The Human Microbiome

Editors

MATTHEW R. PINCUS
ZHIHENG PEI

CLINICS IN LABORATORY MEDICINE

www.labmed.theclinics.com

December 2014 • Volume 34 • Number 4

ELSEVIER

1600 John F. Kennedy Boulevard ● Suite 1800 ● Philadelphia, Pennsylvania, 19103-2899

http://www.theclinics.com

CLINICS IN LABORATORY MEDICINE Volume 34, Number 4
December 2014 ISSN 0272-2712, ISBN-13: 978-0-323-32656-8

Editor: Joanne Husovski
Developmental Editor: Colleen Viola

Reprints. For copies of 100 or more, of articles in this publication, please contact the Commercial Reprints Department, Elsevier Inc., 360 Park Avenue South, New York, New York 10010-1710. Tel. 212-633-3874, Fax: 212-633-3820, E-mail: reprints@elsevier.com.

Clinics in Laboratory Medicine (ISSN 0272-2712) is published quarterly by Elsevier Inc., 360 Park Avenue South, New York, NY 10010-1710. Months of issue are March, June, September, and December. Business and Editorial offices: 1600 John F. Kennedy Blvd., Suite 1800, Philadelphia, PA 19103-2899. Periodicals postage paid at NewYork, NY and additional mailing offices. Subscription prices are $250.00 per year (US individuals), $419.00 per year (US institutions), $135.00 per year (US students), $305.00 per year (Canadian individuals), $510.00 per year (Canadian institutions), $185.00 per year (Canadian students), $390.00 per year (foreign individuals), $510.00 per year (foreign institutions), $185.00 (foreign students). Foreign air speed delivery is included in all Clinics subscription prices. All prices are subject to change without notice. POSTMASTER: Send address changes to *Clinics in Laboratory Medicine*, Elsevier Health Sciences Division, Subscription Customer Service, 3251 Riverport Lane, Maryland Heights, MO 63043. **Customer Service: 1-800-654-2452 (US). From outside of the US and Canada, call 1-314-447-8871. Fax: 1-314-447-8029. E-mail: journalscustomerservice-usa@elsevier.com (for print support) or journalsonlinesupport-usa@elsevier. com (for online support).**

Clinics in Laboratory Medicine is covered in *EMBASE/Exerpta Medica, MEDLINE/PubMed (Index Medicus), Cinahl, Current Contents/Clinical Medicine, BIOSIS and ISI/BIOMED.*

Contributors

EDITORS

MATTHEW R. PINCUS, MD, PhD
Professor of Pathology, SUNY Downstate Medical Center, Brooklyn, New York; Chief, Department of Pathology and Laboratory Medicine, New York Harbor VA Medical Center, New York, New York

ZHIHENG PEI, MD, PhD, FASCP
Associate Professor of Pathology, New York University Medical Center; Staff Physician, Department of Pathology and Laboratory Medicine, New York Harbor VA Medical Center, New York, New York

AUTHORS

JULIAN A. ABRAMS, MD, MS
Florence Irving Assistant Professor of Medicine, Division of Digestive and Liver Diseases, Columbia University Medical Center, New York, New York

JONATHAN BAGHDADI, MD
Clinical Instructor, Department of Medicine, New York University School of Medicine, New York, New York

J. PAUL BROOKS, PhD
Department of Statistical Sciences and Operations Research, Virginia Commonwealth University, Richmond, Virginia

GREGORY A. BUCK, PhD
Department of Microbiology and Immunology, Center for the Study of Biological Complexity, Richmond, Virginia

JANELL CARTER, MD
Resident Physician, Department of Pathology, New York University School of Medicine, New York, New York

THERESA L. CHANG, PhD
Associate Professor, Department of Microbiology and Molecular Genetics, Public Health Research Institute, Rutgers-New Jersey Medical School, Newark, New Jersey

NOAMI CHAUDHARY, MD
Clinical Instructor, Department of Medicine, New York University School of Medicine, New York, New York

MARGARET CHO, MD
Resident Physician, Department of Pathology, New York University School of Medicine, New York, New York

JENNIFER M. FETTWEIS, PhD
Department of Microbiology and Immunology, Center for the Study of Biological Complexity, Richmond, Virginia

DANIEL E. FREEDBERG, MD, MS
Instructor of Medicine, Division of Digestive and Liver Diseases, Columbia University Medical Center, New York, New York

IAN GANLY, MD, PhD
Head and Neck Service, Department of Surgery, Memorial Sloan Kettering Cancer Center, New York, New York

SAUL HARARI, MD
Resident Physician, Department of Pathology, New York University School of Medicine, New York, New York

BERNICE HUANG, PhD
Department of Microbiology and Immunology, Center for the Study of Biological Complexity, Richmond, Virginia

RICHARD H. HUNT, MB, FRCP, FRCPEd, FRCPC, AGAF, MACG, MWGO
Professor Emeritus, Division of Gastroenterology, Department of Medicine, McMaster University Health Science Centre, McMaster University; Farncombe Family Digestive Health Research Institute, Hamilton, Ontario, Canada

KIMBERLY K. JEFFERSON, PhD
Department of Microbiology and Immunology, Center for the Study of Biological Complexity, Richmond, Virginia

HU JIANZHONG, PhD
Assistant Professor, Department of Genetics and Genomic Sciences, Icahn School of Medicine at Mount Sinai, New York, New York

ZAIN KASSAM, MD, MPH, FRCPC
Department of Biological Engineering, Massachusetts Institute of Technology, Cambridge, Massachusetts

BENJAMIN LEBWOHL, MD, MS
Assistant Professor of Medicine and Epidemiology, Division of Digestive and Liver Diseases, Columbia University Medical Center; Celiac Disease Center at Columbia University, New York, New York

CHRISTINE H. LEE, MD, FRCPC, FIDSA
Division of Infectious Diseases, Department of Medicine; Department of Pathology and Molecular Medicine, McMaster University; Hamilton Regional Laboratory Medicine Program, Hamilton, Ontario, Canada

ZHIHENG PEI, MD, PhD, FASCP
Associate Professor of Pathology, New York University Medical Center; Staff Physician, Department of Pathology and Laboratory Medicine, New York Harbor VA Medical Center, New York, New York

JANUARY T. SALAS, PhD
Postdoctoral fellow, Public Health Research Institute, Rutgers-New Jersey Medical School, Newark, New Jersey

LAURA WANG, MBBS
Head and Neck Service, Department of Surgery, Memorial Sloan Kettering Cancer Center, New York, New York

LIYING YANG, MD
Assistant Professor of Medicine, Department of Medicine, New York University School of Medicine, New York, New York

Contents

The cause of colorectal cancer (CRC) is multifactorial, with genetic, molecular, inflammatory, and environmental risk factors. Recently, the gut microbiota has been recognized as a new environmental contributor to CRC in both animal models and human studies. An additional interplay of the gut microbiome with inflammation is also evident in studies that have shown that inflammation alone or the presence of bacteria/bacterial metabolites alone is not enough to promote tumorigenesis. Rather, complex interrelationships with the gut microbiome, inflammation, genetics, and other environmental factors are evident in progression of colorectal tumors.

The role that bacteria play in the etiology and predisposition to cancer is of increasing interest, particularly since the development of high-throughput genetic-based assays. With this technology, it has become possible to comprehensively examine entire microbiomes as a functional entity. This article focuses on the understanding of bacteria and its association with oral squamous cell carcinoma.

With the development of culture-independent technique, a complex microbiome has been established and described in the distal esophagus. The incidence of esophageal adenocarcinoma (EAC) has increased dramatically in the United States. Studies documenting an altered microbiome associated with EAC and its precedents suggest that dysbiosis may be contributing to carcinogenesis, potentially mediated by interactions with toll-like receptors. Investigations attempting to associate viruses with EAC have not been as consistent. Currently available data are cross-sectional and therefore cannot prove causal relationships. Prospectively, microbiome studies open a new avenue to the understanding of the etiology and pathogenesis of reflux disorders and EAC.

Human immunodeficiency virus (HIV) primary infection occurs at mucosa tissues, suggesting an intricate interplay between the microbiome and HIV infection. Recent advanced technologies of high-throughput sequencing and bioinformatics allow researchers to explore nonculturable microbes, including bacteria, virus, and fungi, and their association with diseases. HIV/simian immunodeficiency virus infection is associated with microbiome shifts and immune activation that may affect the outcome of disease progression. In this review, the authors focus on microbiome in HIV infection at various mucosal compartments. Understanding the relationship between microbiome and HIV may offer insights into development of better strategies for HIV prevention and treatment.

Deep sequence analysis of the vaginal microbiome is revealing an unexpected complexity that was not anticipated as recently as several years ago. The lack of clarity in the definition of a healthy vaginal microbiome, much less an unhealthy vaginal microbiome, underscores the need for more investigation of these phenomena. Some clarity may be gained by the careful analysis of the genomes of the specific bacteria in these women. Ongoing studies will clarify this process and offer relief for women with recurring vaginal maladies and hope for pregnant women to avoid the experience of preterm birth.

Extensive genetic studies have identified more than 140 loci predisposing to Crohn disease (CD). Several major CD susceptibility genes have been shown to impair biological function with regard to immune response to recognizing and clearance of bacterial infection. Recent human microbiome studies suggest that the gut microbiome composition is differentiated in carriers of many risk variants of major CD susceptibility genes. This interplay between host genetics and its associated gut microbiome may play an essential role in the pathogenesis of CD. The ongoing microbiome research is aimed to investigate the detailed host genetics-microbiome interacting mechanism.

Potent gastric acid suppression using proton pump inhibitors (PPIs) is common in clinical practice but may have important effects on human health that are mediated through changes in the gastrointestinal microbiome. In the esophagus, PPIs change the normal bacterial milieu to decrease distal esophageal exposure to inflammatory gram-negative bacteria. In the stomach, PPIs alter the abundance and location of gastric *Helicobacter pylori* and other bacteria. In the small bowel, PPIs cause polymicrobial small bowel bacterial overgrowth and have been associated with the diagnosis of celiac disease. In the colon, PPIs associate with incident but not recurrent *Clostridium difficile* infection.

Clostridium difficile infection (CDI) is one of the most common health care–associated infections in the United States. Currently, there are no standardized methods to prepare or deliver the fecal microbiota transplantation (FMT). Various methods are used to prepare the FMT, which is usually administered via nasogastric tube, colonoscopy, or by enema. Several clinical trials are underway to assess the true efficacy and safety of FMT for CDI. These trials include CDI studies assessing FMT via colonoscopy and frozen encapsulation, fresh versus frozen-and-thawed FMT by enema, FMT compared with a vancomycin taper, and FMT in the pediatric population.

CLINICS IN LABORATORY MEDICINE

FORTHCOMING ISSUES

Automated Blood Cell Counters
Carlo Brugnara and Alexander Kratz,
Editors

Diagnostic Testing for Enteric Pathogens
Alexander McAdam and
Collette Fitzgerald, *Editors*

Targeted Therapies
Matthew R. Pincus, *Editor*

The Complement System
Patricia Giclas, *Editor*

RECENT ISSUES

September 2014
Anticoagulants
Jerrold H. Levy, *Editor*

June 2014
Respiratory Infections
Michael J. Loeffelholz, *Editor*

March 2014
Cardiac Markers
Kent B. Lewandrowski, *Editor*

RELATED INTEREST

Gastroenterology Clinics of North America
December 2012 (Vol. 41, Issue. 4, Pages 717–731)
Early Development of Intestinal Microbiota: Implications for Future Health
José M. Saavedra and Anne M. Dattilo, *Authors*
In Clinical Applications of Probiotics in Gastroenterology: Questions and Answers
Gerald Friedman, *Editor*

Preface

Beyond Infectious Disease: Welcome to the Era of Population Microbiology

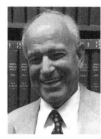 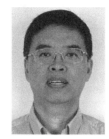

Matthew R. Pincus, MD, PhD   Zhiheng Pei, MD, PhD, FASCP
Editors

The emergence of the germ theory of disease coupled with Robert Koch's famous postulates has shaped nearly all aspects of clinical microbiology since the late nineteenth century and laid the foundation for a new medical discipline: infectious diseases. Under the guidance of the one pathogen-one disease paradigm, many diseases have been demonstrated to have a microbial cause and are classified as infectious diseases. The paradigm also provides essential principles in research and development of specific diagnosis with pathogen isolation and identification, targeted treatment with antibiotics, and effective prevention with vaccines. The development of the infectious disease concept is one of the greatest achievements in public health that alone contributed to a sharp drop in infant and child mortality and to the 29.2-year increase in life expectancy in the twentieth century.[1]

However, the limitation to one pathogen in one disease has sharply narrowed our vision by selecting and focusing on single colonies and ignoring the large majority until the last decade, when the technical advances in high throughput sequencing and bioinformatics made it possible to scrutinize the entire microbial community (microbiota/microbiome) in the human body. Commensal bacteria colonize all mucosal and skin surfaces and outnumber human cells by a factor of 10. During millions of years of mutual hosting, commensal bacteria have evolved into a symbiotic relationship with human hosts, performing essential functions in the development of the immune system, digestion of dietary nutrients beyond our own capability, and prevention of pathogenic bacterial colonization. If these functions are vital to humans, one would expect disturbance to the bacterial population could affect susceptibility of an individual to various diseases. In this special issue dedicated to microbiome in human diseases, eight reviews explore the state of microbiome in a variety of clinical conditions.

The human microbiome recently received heightened attention in cancer research after the landmark discovery that *Helicobacter pylori* induces peptic ulcer and is

Clin Lab Med 34 (2014) xi–xiii
http://dx.doi.org/10.1016/j.cll.2014.09.001
0272-2712/14/$ – see front matter Published by Elsevier Inc.

labmed.theclinics.com

strongly associated with cancer of the stomach and of the association of bacterial microbiota with cancers of the colon, pancreas, mouth, and perhaps the esophagus. In this issue, three reviews summarize the most recent advances in cancer cause in the context of the human microbiome. Drs Cho, Carter, Harari, and Pei discuss the interrelationships of the gut microbiome and inflammation in colorectal carcinogenesis. An important concept has been drawn from animal models of colitis-associated colorectal cancer that inflammation induced by knockout of genes related to immunity or the presence of bacteria and bacterial metabolites is necessary, but each factor alone is not sufficient to promote tumorigenesis, pointing to the need to study both the host genetics and the microbes in colorectal cancer.

Then, Drs Wang and Ganly summarize the oral microbiome in oral cancer. Here, bacteria play roles in the metabolism of chemical carcinogens. In vitro studies have demonstrated that oral commensal bacteria are capable of converting ethanol to acetaldehyde, a recognized carcinogen and activating procarcinogen in cigarette smoke.

Drs Baghdadi, Chaudhary, Pei, and Yang provide a new insight into the cause of the recent surge in the incidence of esophageal adenocarcinoma with the possible role of dysbiosis contributing to carcinogenesis. In the esophagus, bacteria may enhance and maintain chronic inflammation induced by gastroesophageal reflux via triggering activation of the toll-like receptors on the NFκB pathway.

Three reviews further explore the role of microbiome in microbial and inflammatory diseases. Drs Salas and Chang discuss recent findings on microbiome alteration in HIV infection. The review broadly covers multiple mucosal compartments relevant to systemic and local manifestations of HIV infection. With HIV as the known cause of AIDS, study of the microbiome in HIV infection is often aimed at whether the microbiome plays accessory roles in disease acquisition and progression. Microbiome shifts following HIV infection as observed in several recent studies may activate the immune system that promotes viral replication and drives CD4+ T-cell depletion, hence shortening the course to reach the AIDS stage.

Drs Huang, Fettweis, Brooks, Jefferson, and Buck provide us with a changing landscape of the vaginal microbiome. The well-known old school of thought states that healthy vaginal communities are dominated by only one or two *Lactobacillus* species, which inhibit pathogen colonization by lowering the pH through lactic acid production and by competing for nutrients and space. However, deep sequence analysis of the vaginal microbiome is revealing an unexpected complexity. There are several distinct types of communities, and the prevalence of these communities varies significantly among different racial and ethnic groups. While *Lactobacillus* species dominates most healthy women's vaginal microbiome, paradoxically, many women with bacterial vaginosis exhibit homogenous vaginal microbiomes dominated by lactobacilli; *Gardnerella vaginalis*, a signature for bacterial vaginosis, has been found to be the dominant species in the vagina of healthy women, especially in African women. It appears that bacteria with identical 16S rRNA sequences may have vastly different beneficial/pathogenic potentials encoded by genes located outside of the 16S rRNA genes in the genomes.

Dr Hu reviews gut microbiome in Crohn disease (CD) in the context of host genetics. CD has long been suspected to have both genetic and microbial causes but remained a mystery because it does not fit into the paradigm of one gene-one disease or one pathogen-one disease. Single-nucleotide polymorphism profiling now has identified more than 140 loci predisposing to CD and high-throughput sequencing discovered gut microbiome composition associated with carriers of some of the CD susceptibility genes.

Except for food and antibiotics, few exogenous factors are known to cause changes in the human microbiome. In this issue, two reviews explore treatments that affect the gut microbiome in clinical practice. Drs Freedberg, Lebwohl, and Abrams address the impact of proton pump inhibitors (PPIs) on the human gastrointestinal microbiome. PPIs, widely used for the treatment of gastroesophageal reflux and *Helicobacter* gastritis, may alter the gastrointestinal microbiome via suppression of gastric acid secretion, induction of hypergastrinemia and hyperparathyroidism, interference with nutrient absorption, and inhibition of proton pumps of bacteria. Studies have found that PPIs deplete esophageal gram-negative bacteria and facilitate *H pylori* eradication but promote gastric dysbiosis, cause small intestinal bacterial overgrowth, and increase the risk for *Clostridium difficile* infection.

This issue concludes with the review by Drs Kassam, Lee, and Hunt on the emerging treatment of *C difficile* infection with fecal microbiota transplantation and insights into future challenges. It is well-known that *C difficile* infection is caused by alteration of the normal gut microbiota by antibiotics, which remove the resistance to *C difficile* colonization. Restoration of gut microbiome by fecal microbiota transplantation represents one of the most fruitful therapies developed out of translational medicine. This triumph of translational medical research will enable clinical personnel to implement effective therapy for this serious infectious disease.

These reviews discuss specific examples of inflammatory, infectious, and neoplastic diseases. Although these conditions are different, they all involve the human-microbe relationship in the context of the entire bacterial population. Bacterial flora population-based microbiology is introducing a new category of diseases (ie, microbiome diseases or microecological diseases) into clinical practice. Unlike infectious diseases, it can be expected that new diseases would be promoted and/or caused by specific mixes of bacterial community. These diseases, even though caused by multiple bacteria, are not infectious and are not preventable by vaccination. These features render Koch's postulates not suitable for proving cause.

Established methods in clinical microbiology laboratories designed to detect and identify single pathogens such as selective media and colony picking or even specific PCR could be replaced by high-throughput but low-cost sequencing technologies to allow the detection of specific pathogens for the diagnosis of infectious diseases as well as profiling the entire microbial population for microbiome diseases or microecological diseases.

This work was supported in part by the Department of Veterans Affairs, Veterans Health Administration, Office of Research and Development and grants U01CA18237, UH3CA140233, R01AI110372, R01CA159036, R21ES023421, and R03CA159414 from the National Institutes of Health (NIH) and NIH Human Microbiome Project.

Matthew R. Pincus, MD, PhD
SUNY Downstate Medical Center
450 Clarkson Avenue
Brooklyn, NY 11203, USA

Zhiheng Pei, MD, PhD, FASCP
New York University Medical Center
550 First Avenue
New York, NY 10016, USA

E-mail addresses:
Matthew.Pincus2@va.gov (M.R. Pincus)
zhiheng.pei@va.gov (Z. Pei)

REFERENCE

1. Center for Disease Control and Prevention. Achievements in public health, 1900–1999: control of infectious diseases. MMWR 1999;48:621–9.

The Interrelationships of the Gut Microbiome and Inflammation in Colorectal Carcinogenesis

Margaret Cho, MD[a], Janell Carter, MD[a], Saul Harari, MD[a],
Zhiheng Pei, MD, PhD, FASCP[a,b,c,*]

KEYWORDS

- Gut microbiome • Colorectal cancer • Inflammation • Carcinogenesis

KEY POINTS

- The cause of colorectal cancer (CRC) is multifactorial with genetic, molecular, inflammatory, and environmental risk factors. Recently, the gut microbiota has been recognized as a new environmental contributor to CRC in both animal models and human studies.
- An additional interplay of the gut microbiome with inflammation is also evident in studies that have shown that inflammation alone or the presence of bacteria/bacterial metabolites alone is not enough to promote tumorigenesis.
- Complex interrelationships with the gut microbiome, inflammation, genetics, and other environmental factors are evident in progression of colorectal tumors.

INTRODUCTION

The last decade has brought a revolution in the understanding of microorganisms vis-à-vis their environment/mammalian hosts. These radical changes in thought not only challenge ideas that dominated biological and medical sciences for more than a hundred years but at a visceral level call, into question the definition of the human identity. The emergence of the germ theory of disease in the late nineteenth century,

Disclosure: The authors have nothing to disclose.
This work was supported in part by grants U01CA18237, UH3CA140233, R01CA159036, and R03CA159414 from the National Cancer Institute and NIH Human Microbiome Project, and by the Department of Veterans Affairs, Veterans Health Administration, Office of Research and Development.
[a] Department of Pathology, New York University School of Medicine, 560 First Avenue, New York, NY 10016, USA; [b] Department of Medicine, New York University School of Medicine, 560 First Avenue, New York, NY 10016, USA; [c] Department of Veterans Affairs New York Harbor Healthcare System, 423 East 23rd Street, Room 6030W, New York, NY 10010, USA
* Corresponding author. Veterans Affairs Medical Center, 423 East 23rd Street, Room 6030W, New York, NY 10010.
E-mail address: zhiheng.pei@med.nyu.edu

highlighted by the propagation of Robert Koch's famous postulates, and the ensuing discovery of antibiotics some decades later, exemplify the view of microorganism as a foreign other, with disease-causing potential (pathogens) that often needs to be treated via medical eradication. In the common parlance, germs are bad and not to be spread. Although there was a movement recognizing the potential for bacteria to benefit their host (probiotics) during the twentieth century, it is only in the last decade or so that the true extent, complexity, and intimacy of this relationship have taken form.

It is now generally accepted that bacteria are (critical to their ecosystems) ubiquitous and colonizers of all exposed human body surfaces, including the entire alimentary tract. Bacterial organisms living in/on a human host outnumber that host's native cells by a factor of 10. These bacterial communities (microbiota) become a part of us from birth and participate in what is now regarded as a relationship of symbiotic mutualism, whereby the human provides a nutrient-enriched tailored living environment. In return, bacteria play a critical role for the health and development of the human species. There is evidence, for example, that the presence of the bacterial microbiome is integral for modulation of the human immune system, digestion of dietary nutrients otherwise impervious to human enzymes, and prevention of pathogenic bacterial disease. Given these observations, some go as far as to characterize the human and their corresponding microbiota as parts of a vastly greater superorganism. At a minimum, it is clear that mammals and microorganisms have coevolved to produce an intricate and vital symbiotic relationship.

Reminiscent of the inextricable linkage between the invention/popularization of the microscope and the discovery of microorganisms, both attributed to Van Leeuwenhoek (late seventeenth century), the recent charge to characterize whole populations of bacteria and viruses was permitted by advances in experimental techniques and laboratory sciences. These advances include advancements in bioinformatics, biological analytics, and DNA/RNA collection and sequencing techniques, which allow for high throughput approaches to specify and quantitate myriads of different bacteria. Although a single strain of bacteria may be held accountable as an etiologically specific cause for diseases, such as *Clostridium difficile* for pseudomembranous colitis, perhaps the more pertinent question is: what changes in the usually protective microbiome (dysbiosis) allowed for such infection? In that example, the answer is antibiotic-induced dysbiosis. Moreover, the state of microbiota has been associated with conditions such as diabetes, skin disease, obesity, inflammatory bowel disease (IBD), and even cancer, all of which are commonly regarded as noninfectious processes.

Although inflammatory, infectious, and neoplastic diseases are often considered categorically distinct processes, evidence has shown significant overlap between them. It is estimated that 15% of worldwide cancer is of infectious nature, with human papillomavirus, hepatitis B virus, hepatitis C virus, human herpesvirus 8, and *Helicobacter pylori* recognized as the definitive cause of cervical cancer, liver cancer, Kaposi sarcoma, and stomach cancer/lymphoma, respectively. Furthermore, direct causation of cancer by chronic inflammatory conditions is well documented. The association of IBD with increased risk of colon cancer is a case in point. Thus, it should come as no surprise that alterations of the microbiome may lead to infectious, inflammatory, and cancerous disease. The focus of this review is to detail the interrelationship between colorectal cancer (CRC) and the gut microbiome.

BACKGROUND

CRC is the second leading type of cancer in females and the third in males worldwide, with more than 1.2 million new cases and more than 600,000 estimated deaths in

2008.[1] In the United States, an estimate of 142,820 new cases of CRC with more than 50,000 deaths occur annually.[2] However, both incidence and mortality of CRC in the United States have steadily declined, and this decrease may be attributed to prevention, early screening, detection, and treatment of CRC.[3]

Major risk factors of CRC have also been established. In sporadic CRC, age is a risk factor with increased incidence between the ages of 40 and 50 years and with 90% of cases occurring after the age of 50 years.[4] In the United States, men have a 25% higher incidence of CRC than women, and African Americans have a 20% higher incidence than whites.

Genetic risk factors are evident in hereditary CRC syndromes such as familial adenomatous polyposis (FAP) and hereditary nonpolyposis CRC (HNPCC). In FAP, the adenomatous polyposis coli (APC) gene located on chromosome 5 is mutated and accounts for less than 1% of CRCs.[5] HNPCC accounts for 3% to 5% of CRCs and has a germline mutation in one allele of a mismatch repair gene, including hMLH1, hMSH2, hMSH6, or PMS2, with inactivation of the second allele by loss of heterozygosity, somatic mutation, or promoter hypermethylation.[5,6] HNPCC-related CRCs present with KRAS mutations and do not have BRAF mutations.[7] Additional risk factors include personal or family history of CRC or adenomatous colon polyps (**Fig. 1**).[8,9]

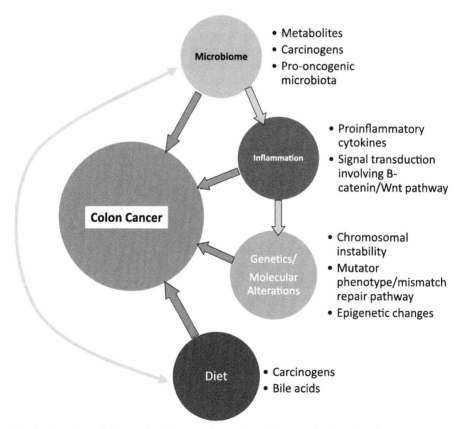

- Metabolites
- Carcinogens
- Pro-oncogenic microbiota

- Proinflammatory cytokines
- Signal transduction involving B-catenin/Wnt pathway

- Chromosomal instability
- Mutator phenotype/mismatch repair pathway
- Epigenetic changes

- Carcinogens
- Bile acids

Fig. 1. Overview of factors leading to colorectal carcinogenesis. The microbiome interacts with inflammatory mechanisms as well as dietary factors in progression of tumorigenesis.

Most CRCs are sporadic, with tumorigenesis that involves mutations in APC (5q), DNA hypomethylation, and acquisition of multiple additional alterations, especially in KRAS2 (12p), DCC (18q), and p53 (17p).[10,11] BRAF mutations are especially prevalent in sporadic CRC of smokers.[12]

At least 3 molecular pathways have been outlined in colorectal tumorigenesis. The chromosomal instability pathway is seen in FAP as well as in sporadic CRC and is characterized by chromosomal abnormalities, including deletions, insertions, and loss of heterozygosity.[13] The mutator phenotype/mismatch repair pathway is represented by HNPCC, as outlined earlier. The third hypermethylation phenotype, hyperplastic/serrated polyp pathway, includes epigenetic changes, including hypermethylation of some CpG islands. This alteration may result in hypermethylation of the promoter region of mismatch repair enzymes such as MLH1.[14]

IBD including ulcerative colitis (UC) and Crohn disease also predispose to CRC. Although the pathogenesis of CRC in the setting of IBD is poorly understood, studies suggest that there are differences from sporadic CRC. In contrast to sporadic CRC, mutations in the ras proto-oncogene are less frequently observed in CRC associated with UC and occur as a late event.[15–17] In CRC associated with IBD, loss of heterozygosity for p53 and SRC activation occur earlier.[15,17]

In addition to genetic factors, environmental factors also predispose individuals to CRC. In particular, diet has been linked to CRC. Some studies have shown that high intake of red and processed meats, highly refined grains and starches, sugars, fat, and alcohol are associated with an increased risk of CRC.[18,19]

Microorganisms such as bacteria have been suggested as links to CRC. One example is the association of *Streptococcus bovis* with CRC, which has been previously recognized.[20] However, the cause of this association is unclear. The gut microbiota is an emerging environmental contributor to CRC, which has led to various investigations in both animal and human models, which are further discussed.

NORMAL BACTERIAL MICROBIOTA

The colon contains an estimated load of 10^{13} to 10^{14} microorganisms, which are composed of more than 1000 different bacterial species.[21,22] These microorganisms collectively comprise the microbiota.[23,24] The normal colonic microbiota includes anaerobes such as *Bacteroides*, *Eubacterium*, *Bifidobacterium*, *Fusobacterium*, *Peptostreptococcus*, and *Atopobium*.[24,25] Facultative anaerobes include Lactobacilli, Enterococci, Streptococci, and Enterobacteriaceae and are present at approximately 1000-fold lower levels.[24] However, the number and variability of bacterial species among individuals remain to be characterized.[24,26]

MICROBIOTA AND CARCINOGENESIS IN THE COLON

The population of microbiota in healthy adults is relatively stable over time, with fluctuations occurring in response to environmental and pathologic events.[24,27] An association between colon cancer and specific bacterial species, including *Streptococcus bovis*, *Bacteroides*, and *Clostridium*, has been established.[24,28–30] Other bacterial strains such as *Lactobacillus acidophilus* and *Bifidobacterium longum* have been shown to inhibit tumorigenesis.[24,31,32] Hence, the microbiota seems to be a balance between beneficial and harmful bacteria, with shifts influencing carcinogenesis.

Adherent/invasive *Escherichia coli* strains were abundant in the colonic mucosa of patients with CRC and adenoma but not in those with normal colonic mucosa.[33] Other studies have reported microbiome maps generated from late-stage CRC tissue. A relative abundance of Bacteroidaceae, Streptococcaceae, Fusobacteriaceae,

Peptostreptococcaceae, Veillonellaceae, and Pasteurellaceae and a significantly lower level of Lachnospiraceae, Ruminococcaceae, and Lactobacillaceae have been found in cancerous tissues compared with the intestinal lumen.[24,34] Chen and colleagues[34] examined 16S rRNA genes to profile the microbiota present in patients with CRC compared with healthy control individuals and found considerable differences between the 2 groups. The mucosa-adherent microbiota, *Bifidobacterium*, *Faecalibacterium*, and *Blautia*, were reduced in patients with CRC, whereas *Porphyromonas* and *Mogibacterium* were enriched.[24] In the lumen, Erysipelotrichaceae, Prevotellaceae, and Coriobacteriaceae were also increased in patients with CRC, which suggests that intestinal lumen microflora increases risk for CRC through direct interactions with the host.[24,34]

In a study by Gueimonde and colleagues,[35] quantitative reverse transcriptase polymerase chain reaction was used to analyze colonic mucosa samples obtained from 21 patients with CRC, 9 patients with diverticulitis, and 4 patients with IBD. The CRC patients had significantly lower levels of *B longum* and *Bifidobacterium bifidum* when compared with the other patients. In a study by Shen and colleagues,[36] sequencing of 335 clones for phylogenetic and taxonomic analyses of adherent bacteria present in 21 patients with adenoma and 23 individuals who did not have adenoma showed higher numbers of *Proteobacteria* and lower numbers of *Bacteroidetes* in patients with adenoma. Sobhani and colleagues[37] analyzed stool bacterial DNA using pyrosequencing and subsequent principal component analysis to detect shifts in the composition of the microbiota of patients with CRC and found *Bacteroides/Prevotella* species to be more abundant in patients who have cancer than in control individuals. These studies show a complex association of gut microbiota with CRC development.

Fusobacterium, a gram-negative anaerobe that is often associated with periodontal disease,[38] has received heightened attention recently after several groups reported its link to CRC. Early studies showed that *Fusobacterium* is more abundant in human CRC tissue than in adjacent normal tissue,[39,40] but a late study found that even in normal rectal mucosa, *Fusobacterium* is enriched in CRC case patients compared with control individuals.[34] The difference is also evident in stool samples.[41,42] The enrichment of *Fusobacterium* can also be identified in colorectal adenoma, the precursor of CRC.[42,43] Patients with CRC with high fusobacterial levels had a significantly longer overall survival time than patients with low and moderate levels of the bacterium.[42] CRC with a high level of *Fusobacterium* is associated with CpG island methylator phenotype, TP53 wild-type, hMLH1 methylation positivity, microsatellite instability, and CHD7/8 mutation.[44] FadA adhesin of *Fusobacterium* can mediate bacterial adherence and invasion and induce oncogenic and inflammatory responses to stimulate growth of CRC cells by activation of β-catenin signaling via FadA binding to E-cadherin.[45]

Several animal studies have shown bacterial strains to be implicated in colorectal carcinogenesis. The first reported link between the gut microbiota and CRC development was in 1975 by Reddy and colleagues,[46] who reported that 93% of conventionally maintained rats developed chemically induced CRC and only 20% of germ-free rats developed CRC. In carcinogen-treated rats, *Streptococcus bovis* and its antigens extracted from the bacterial cell wall led to increased expression of proliferation markers and formation of aberrant, hyperproliferative colonic crypts.[24,47]

Animal studies have also shown a link between the effects of the microbiota on metabolites and progression to CRC. Many carcinogenic compounds are metabolized in the liver and then conjugated to glucuronic acid before being excreted via the bile into the small intestine.[24] In the colon, bacterial β-glucuronidase hydrolyzes the conjugates and releases the parent compound and activated metabolite.[48] One example is seen with the colon carcinogen, dimethylhydrazine (DMH), which is metabolized in the liver. Small amounts of the procarcinogenic conjugate of the activated metabolite, methylazoxymethanol, are excreted in the bile and released in the colon through hydrolysis by bacteria.[49] Germ-free animals treated with DMH had fewer colon tumors when compared with conventional animals, and microflora-derived β-glucuronidase played an important role in the cause of CRC.[24,49]

Intestinal microbiota also play an important role in the metabolism of bile acids. The process of 7α-dehydroxylation involves the conversion of cholic to deoxycholic acid (DCA) and chenodeoxycholic to lithocholic acid.[24,50] In an animal model, infusion of DCA caused intestinal mucosal damage and led to increase in cell proliferation,[51] and DCA-induced DNA damage also triggered calcium ion–dependent apoptosis independent of p53.[24,52] In a rat model, the capacity for DCA to enhance colon tumor development was shown to be attenuated by all-trans retinoic acid.[53] Secondary bile acids may also lead to progression of CRC by supporting apoptosis-resistant cells or by mediating interactions with important secondary messenger signaling systems known to be activated in CRC.[24,54]

Enterotoxigenic *Bacteroides fragilis* (ETBF) belongs to a group of bacterial drivers of CRC that are defined as intestinal bacteria with procarcinogenic features that may initiate CRC development.[24] One mechanism for this process involves the production of DNA-damaging compounds.[24,55] For example, certain *E coli* strains that harbor a polyketide synthetase island, which encodes a genotoxin called colibactin, can induce single-strand DNA breaks and lead to tumorigenesis.[24,55]

Furthermore, gut microbiota also seems to induce chronic inflammation and generate reactive metabolites and carcinogens, leading to development of CRC.[56]

Several experimental models have been used to study the role of microorganisms during the development of inflammation and CRC. ETBF can secrete a *B fragilis* toxin, which can cause human inflammatory diarrhea and stimulate cleavage of the tumor suppressor protein, E-cadherin.[57] Loss of membrane-associated E-cadherin in HT29/C1 cells triggers the nuclear localization of β-catenin, which then binds with T-cell factor-dependent transcriptional activators to induce expression of c-Myc and cyclin D1, which results in persistent cell proliferation.[24,58]

A mouse model of ETBF-induced colitis and carcinogenesis showed enhanced tumorigenesis through induction of infiltration of the lamina propria by interleukin 17 (IL-17)-producing CD4+ T cells (Th17) and γδ-T cells via STAT3 signaling.[24,59] IL-17 can also promote tumor growth in vitro and in vivo via the production of IL-6 by IL-17 receptor-bearing tumor cell lines.[60] Both nuclear factor κB (NF-κB)[61] and STAT-3[62] are key mediators of inflammation-driven carcinogenesis via their putative antiapoptotic and cell cycle activity in colonic epithelial cells and their promotion of procarcinogenic mediators by immune cells.[24]

MICROBIOTA AND INFLAMMATION IN THE COLON

An inflammatory microenvironment has long been associated with contributing to and increasing the risk of CRC. The prototypical IBDs, Crohn disease and UC, both carry an increased risk of malignancy.[63] The interplay between the gut microbiome and inflammation is complex, mainly because there are several microorganisms implicated acting either singly, concurrently, or synergistically. These microorganisms interact with a complex immune system of which several cytokines, chemokines, factors, proteins, and cells are implicated in contributing to setting the stage for tumorigenesis.

Chronic inflammation alters the microenvironment in several ways. It sustains an environment that promotes DNA damage of epithelial cells by introducing and maintaining the presence of nitric oxide and other reactive oxygen species. The cytokines and chemokines produced by inflammatory cells, in response to a microorganism or a by-product of its metabolism, act to eliminate the threat and suppress the immune response against cells undergoing transformation. These factors include nitric oxide, tumor necrosis factor α (TNF-α), IL-1, IL-8, and prostaglandin 2 derivatives, as well as several molecules triggered in the inflammatory signaling pathway. Cytokines and chemokines also enhance tumor survival by promoting angiogenesis. Chief factors include TNF-α, IL-6, and IL-1. The transformation of epithelial cells is modulated by both groups of factors.

Inflammation alone or the presence of bacteria/bacterial metabolites alone is not enough to promote tumorigenesis. As an example, a series of experiments by Joshua and colleagues in which IL-10$^{-/-}$ mice exposed to procarcinogenic compound azoxymethane (AOM) developed colitis and CRC, whereas wild-type mice were colitis free and developed only low-grade dysplasia.[64] Intestinal bacteria are needed to metabolically activate AOM[65] and trigger IL-10 production.[66,67] These experiments support a mechanism of tumorigenesis in which induced chronic inflammation (by the microbiota) and disruption of the balance between proinflammatory and tolerogenic mediators promote disease.

In sporadic cases of CRC and experimental models of colitis-associated cancer, the inducible mediator of prostaglandin synthesis, cyclooxygenase 2 (COX-2), is upregulated.[68,69] The protumorogenic effects of COX-2 upregulation lies in the synthesis of prostaglandin E_2 (PGE$_2$).[70–73] PGE$_2$ also promotes tumor survival and proliferation via β-catenin–dependent signaling. COX-2 inhibits apoptosis by increasing Bcl-2 expression via MAP-kinase or PI3K/AKT signaling pathways.[74–76] It also enhances tumor survival by inducing production of the proangiogenic factors vascular endothelial growth factor and basic fibroblast growth factor.[77]

PROBIOTIC EFFECTS ON CARCINOGENESIS

The use of diet to alter the intestinal microbiota can be seen in the example of probiotics. Probiotics are defined as live microorganisms that confer a health benefit to the host when administered in adequate amounts.[78] Species include *Lactobacillus rhamnosus*, *Lactobacillus reuteri*, and *Lactobacillus acidophilus*.[24] Probiotic mechanisms include immunologic modulation, providing bioactive metabolites, binding mutagens, inhibition of intestinal bacterial enzymes, competition for limited nutrients, inhibition of harmful bacterial mucosa adherence, and inhibition of epithelial cell invasion.[79,80] Molecular mechanisms involve macrophage activation, blocking of cytochrome P450, a reduction in carcinogen generation, downregulation of Ras-p21 expression, promotion of cell differentiation, inhibition of COX-2 upregulation, inhibition of nitric oxide synthase, an increase in short-chain fatty acid production, and a reduction in intestinal pH because of a decrease in the number of putrefactive bacteria.[24,79,81]

Corthesy and colleagues[82] summarized several studies that reported that ingested probiotic strains may persist for short periods and do not become permanent members of the normal microbiota. However, there are benefits, because various studies have shown antiproliferative effects of probiotic species in certain cancer cell lines.[83–85] In particular, Kim and colleagues[85] assessed the anticancer activity and bacterial enzyme inhibition of *Bifidobacterium adolescentis* SPM0212 in human colon cancer cell lines. This strain also was found to inhibit harmful fecal enzymes, including β-glucuronidase, β-glucosidase, tryptophanase, and urease.[85] However, there is a need for more well-controlled clinical studies to elucidate therapeutic and preventive effects of probiotics in various diseases. Even so, the beneficial effects of certain probiotics have been documented in treatment of pouchitis, traveler, and antibiotic-associated diarrhea, irritable bowel syndrome, and rotavirus enteritis.[24,86]

REFERENCES

1. Jemal A, Bray F, Center MM, et al. Global cancer statistics. CA Cancer J Clin 2011;61(2):69–90.
2. Siegel R, Naishadham D, Jemal A. Cancer statistics, 2013. CA Cancer J Clin 2013;63(1):11–30.
3. Kohler BA, Ward E, McCarthy BJ, et al. Annual report to the nation on the status of cancer, 1975-2007, featuring tumors of the brain and other nervous system. J Natl Cancer Inst 2011;103(9):714–36.
4. Eddy DM. Screening for colorectal cancer. Ann Intern Med 1990;113(5):373–84.
5. Burt RW, DiSario JA, Cannon-Albright L. Genetics of colon cancer: impact of inheritance on colon cancer risk. Annu Rev Med 1995;46:371–9.
6. Lynch HT, Smyrk TC, Watson P, et al. Genetics, natural history, tumor spectrum, and pathology of hereditary nonpolyposis colorectal cancer: an updated review. Gastroenterology 1993;104(5):1535–49.
7. Domingo E, Niessen RC, Oliveira C, et al. BRAF-V600E is not involved in the colorectal tumorigenesis of HNPCC in patients with functional MLH1 and MSH2 genes. Oncogene 2005;24(24):3995–8.
8. Atkin WS, Morson BC, Cuzick J. Long-term risk of colorectal cancer after excision of rectosigmoid adenomas. N Engl J Med 1992;326(10):658–62.
9. Imperiale TF, Ransohoff DF. Risk for colorectal cancer in persons with a family history of adenomatous polyps: a systematic review. Ann Intern Med 2012;156(10):703–9.
10. Potter JD. Colorectal cancer: molecules and populations. J Natl Cancer Inst 1999;91(11):916–32.
11. Glei M, Latunde-Dada GO, Klinder A, et al. Iron-overload induces oxidative DNA damage in the human colon carcinoma cell line HT29 clone 19A. Mutat Res 2002;519(1–2):151–61.
12. Samowitz WS, Albertsen H, Sweeney C, et al. Association of smoking, CpG island methylator phenotype, and V600E BRAF mutations in colon cancer. J Natl Cancer Inst 2006;98(23):1731–8.
13. Fearon ER, Vogelstein B. A genetic model for colorectal tumorigenesis. Cell 1990;61(5):759–67.
14. Weisenberger DJ, Siegmund KD, Campan M, et al. CpG island methylator phenotype underlies sporadic microsatellite instability and is tightly associated with BRAF mutation in colorectal cancer. Nat Genet 2006;38(7):787–93.
15. Vogelstein B, Fearon ER, Hamilton SR, et al. Genetic alterations during colorectal-tumor development. N Engl J Med 1988;319(9):525–32.
16. Burmer GC, Levine DS, Kulander BG, et al. c-Ki-ras mutations in chronic ulcerative colitis and sporadic colon carcinoma. Gastroenterology 1990;99(2):416–20.
17. Itzkowitz SH. Inflammatory bowel disease and cancer. Gastroenterol Clin North Am 1997;26(1):129–39.
18. Chan AT, Giovannucci EL. Primary prevention of colorectal cancer. Gastroenterology 2010;138(6):2029–43.

19. Bingham SA. Epidemiology and mechanisms relating diet to risk of colorectal cancer. Nutr Res Rev 1996;9(1):197–239.
20. McIllmurray MB, Langman MJ. Large bowel cancer: causation and management. Gut 1975;16(10):815–20.
21. Arthur JC, Jobin C. The complex interplay between inflammation, the microbiota and colorectal cancer. Gut Microbes 2013;4(3):253–8.
22. Sobhani I, Amiot A, Le Baleur Y, et al. Microbial dysbiosis and colon carcinogenesis: could colon cancer be considered a bacteria-related disease? Therap Adv Gastroenterol 2013;6(3):215–29.
23. Savage DC. Microbial ecology of the gastrointestinal tract. Annu Rev Microbiol 1977;31:107–33.
24. Zhu Q, Gao R, Wu W, et al. The role of gut microbiota in the pathogenesis of colorectal cancer. Tumour Biol 2013;34(3):1285–300.
25. Tlaskalová-Hogenová H, Stepánková R, Hudcovic T, et al. Commensal bacteria (normal microflora), mucosal immunity and chronic inflammatory and autoimmune diseases. Immunol Lett 2004;93(2–3):97–108.
26. Mai V. Dietary modification of the intestinal microbiota. Nutr Rev 2004;62(6 Pt 1): 235–42.
27. Stanghellini V, Barbara G, Cremon C, et al. Gut microbiota and related diseases: clinical features. Intern Emerg Med 2010;5(Suppl 1):S57–63.
28. Gold JS, Bayar S, Salem RR. Association of *Streptococcus bovis* bacteremia with colonic neoplasia and extracolonic malignancy. Arch Surg 2004;139(7):760–5.
29. Moore WE, Moore LH. Intestinal floras of populations that have a high risk of colon cancer. Appl Environ Microbiol 1995;61(9):3202–7.
30. Nakamura J, Kubota Y, Miyaoka M, et al. Comparison of 4 microbial enzymes in *Clostridia* and *Bacteroides* isolated from human feces. Microbiol Immunol 2002; 46(7):487–90.
31. McIntosh GH, Royle PJ, Playne MJ. A probiotic strain of *L. acidophilus* reduces DMH-induced large intestinal tumors in male Sprague-Dawley rats. Nutr Cancer 1999;35(2):153–9.
32. Rowland IR, Bearne CA, Fischer R, et al. The effect of lactulose on DNA damage induced by DMH in the colon of human flora-associated rats. Nutr Cancer 1996; 26(1):37–47.
33. Cuevas-Ramos G, Petit CR, Marcq I, et al. *Escherichia coli* induces DNA damage in vivo and triggers genomic instability in mammalian cells. Proc Natl Acad Sci U S A 2010;107(25):11537–42.
34. Chen W, Liu F, Ling Z, et al. Human intestinal lumen and mucosa-associated microbiota in patients with colorectal cancer. PLoS One 2012;7(6):e39743.
35. Gueimonde M, Ouwehand A, Huhtinen H, et al. Qualitative and quantitative analyses of the bifidobacterial microbiota in the colonic mucosa of patients with colorectal cancer, diverticulitis and inflammatory bowel disease. World J Gastroenterol 2007;13(29):3985–9.
36. Shen XJ, Rawls JF, Randall T, et al. Molecular characterization of mucosal adherent bacteria and associations with colorectal adenomas. Gut Microbes 2010;1(3):138–47.
37. Sobhani I, Tap J, Roudot-Thoraval F, et al. Microbial dysbiosis in colorectal cancer (CRC) patients. PLoS One 2011;6(1):e16393.
38. Signat B, Roques C, Poulet P, et al. *Fusobacterium nucleatum* in periodontal health and disease. Curr Issues Mol Biol 2011;13(2):25–36.
39. Kostic AD, Gevers D, Pedamallu CS, et al. Genomic analysis identifies association of *Fusobacterium* with colorectal carcinoma. Genome Res 2012;22(2):292–8.

40. Castellarin M, Warren RL, Freeman JD, et al. *Fusobacterium nucleatum* infection is prevalent in human colorectal carcinoma. Genome Res 2012;22(2):299–306.
41. Ahn J, Sinha R, Pei Z, et al. Human gut microbiome and risk for colorectal cancer. J Natl Cancer Inst 2013;105(24):1907–11.
42. Flanagan L, Schmid J, Ebert M, et al. *Fusobacterium nucleatum* associates with stages of colorectal neoplasia development, colorectal cancer and disease outcome. Eur J Clin Microbiol Infect Dis 2014;33(8):1381–90.
43. McCoy AN, Araújo-Pérez F, Azcárate-Peril A, et al. *Fusobacterium* is associated with colorectal adenomas. PLoS One 2013;8(1):e53653.
44. Tahara T, Yamamoto E, Suzuki H, et al. *Fusobacterium* in colonic flora and molecular features of colorectal carcinoma. Cancer Res 2014;74(5):1311–8.
45. Rubinstein MR, Wang X, Liu W, et al. *Fusobacterium nucleatum* promotes colorectal carcinogenesis by modulating E-cadherin/β-catenin signaling via its FadA adhesin. Cell Host Microbe 2013;14(2):195–206.
46. Reddy BS, Mastromarino A, Wynder EL. Further leads on metabolic epidemiology of large bowel cancer. Cancer Res 1975;35(11 Pt 2):3403–6.
47. Ellmerich S, Djouder N, Schöller M, et al. Production of cytokines by monocytes, epithelial and endothelial cells activated by *Streptococcus bovis*. Cytokines 2000;12(1):26–31.
48. Rowland IR. The role of the gastrointestinal microbiota in colorectal cancer. Curr Pharm Des 2009;15(13):1524–7.
49. Gill CI, Rowland IR. Diet and cancer: assessing the risk. Br J Nutr 2002; 88(Suppl 1):S73–87.
50. de Giorgio R, Blandizzi C. Targeting enteric neuroplasticity: diet and bugs as new key factors. Gastroenterology 2010;138(5):1663–6.
51. Rubin DC, Shaker A, Levin MS. Chronic intestinal inflammation: inflammatory bowel disease and colitis-associated colon cancer. Front Immunol 2012; 3:107.
52. Powolny A, Xu J, Loo G. Deoxycholate induces DNA damage and apoptosis in human colon epithelial cells expressing either mutant or wild-type p53. Int J Biochem Cell Biol 2001;33(2):193–203.
53. Narahara H, Tatsuta M, Iishi H, et al. K-ras point mutation is associated with enhancement by deoxycholic acid of colon carcinogenesis induced by azoxymethane, but not with its attenuation by all-trans-retinoic acid. Int J Cancer 2000;88(2):157–61.
54. Radley S, Davis AE, Imray CH, et al. Biliary bile acid profiles in familial adenomatous polyposis. Br J Surg 1992;79(1):89–90.
55. Nougayrède JP, Homburg S, Taieb F, et al. *Escherichia coli* induces DNA double-strand breaks in eukaryotic cells. Science 2006;313(5788):848–51.
56. Hope ME, Hold GL, Kain R, et al. Sporadic colorectal cancer–role of the commensal microbiota. FEMS Microbiol Lett 2005;244(1):1–7.
57. Rhee KJ, Wu S, Wu X, et al. Induction of persistent colitis by a human commensal, enterotoxigenic *Bacteroides fragilis*, in wild-type C57BL/6 mice. Infect Immun 2009;77(4):1708–18.
58. Wu S, Morin PJ, Maouyo D, et al. *Bacteroides fragilis* enterotoxin induces c-Myc expression and cellular proliferation. Gastroenterology 2003;124(2):392–400.
59. Wu S, Rhee KJ, Albesiano E, et al. A human colonic commensal promotes colon tumorigenesis via activation of T helper type 17 T cell responses. Nat Med 2009; 15(9):1016–22.
60. Wang L, Yi T, Kortylewski M, et al. IL-17 can promote tumor growth through an IL-6-Stat3 signaling pathway. J Exp Med 2009;206(7):1457–64.

61. Karin M. Nuclear factor-kappaB in cancer development and progression. Nature 2006;441(7092):431–6.
62. Yu H, Kortylewski M, Pardoll D. Crosstalk between cancer and immune cells: role of STAT3 in the tumour microenvironment. Nat Rev Immunol 2007;7(1):41–51.
63. Moossavi S, Bishehsari F. Inflammation in sporadic colorectal cancer. Arch Iran Med 2012;15(3):166–70.
64. Uronis JM, Mühlbauer M, Herfarth HH, et al. Modulation of the intestinal microbiota alters colitis associated colorectal cancer susceptibility. PLoS One 2009; 4(6):e6026.
65. Neufert C, Becker C, Neurath MF. An inducible mouse model of colon carcinogenesis for the analysis of sporadic and inflammation-driven tumor progression. Nat Protoc 2007;2:1998–2004.
66. Ivanov II, Frutos Rde L, Manel N, et al. Specific microbiota direct the differentiation of IL-17-producing T-helper cells in the mucosa of the small intestine. Cell Host Microbe 2008;4:337–49.
67. Mazmanian SK, Round JL, Kasper DL. A microbial symbiosis factor prevents intestinal inflammatory disease. Nature 2008;453(7195):620–5.
68. Sheehan KM, Sheahan K, O'Donoghue DP, et al. The relationship between cyclooxygenase-2 expression and colorectal cancer. JAMA 1999;282(13): 1254–7.
69. Arber N, Eagle CJ, Spicak J, et al. Celecoxib for the prevention of colorectal adenomatous polyps. N Engl J Med 2006;355(9):885–95.
70. Taketo MM. COX-2 and colon cancer. Inflamm Res 1998;47(Suppl 2):S112–6.
71. Pugh S, Thomas GA. Patients with adenomatous polyps and carcinomas have increased colonic mucosal prostaglandin E2. Gut 1994;35(5):675–8.
72. Yang VW, Shields JM, Hamilton SR, et al. Size-dependent increase in prostanoid levels in adenomas of patients with familial adenomatous polyposis. Cancer Res 1998;58(8):1750–3.
73. Kawamori T, Uchiya N, Sugimura T, et al. Enhancement of colon carcinogenesis by prostaglandin E2 administration. Carcinogenesis 2003;24(5):985–90.
74. Castellone MD, Teramoto H, Williams BO, et al. Prostaglandin E2 promotes colon cancer cell growth through a Gs-axin-beta-catenin signaling axis. Science 2005;310(5753):1504–10.
75. Tessner TG, Muhale F, Riehl TE, et al. Prostaglandin E2 reduces radiation-induced epithelial apoptosis through a mechanism involving AKT activation and bax translocation. J Clin Invest 2004;114(11):1676–85.
76. Pozzi A, Yan X, Macias-Perez I, et al. Colon carcinoma cell growth is associated with prostaglandin E2/EP4 receptor-evoked ERK activation. J Biol Chem 2004; 279(28):29797–804.
77. Tsujii M, Kawano S, DuBois RN. Cyclooxygenase-2 expression in human colon cancer cells increases metastatic potential. Proc Natl Acad Sci U S A 1997; 94(7):3336–40.
78. Zhu Y, Michelle Luo T, Jobin C, et al. Gut microbiota and probiotics in colon tumorigenesis. Cancer Lett 2011;309(2):119–27.
79. Pala V, Sieri S, Berrino F, et al. Yogurt consumption and risk of colorectal cancer in the Italian European prospective investigation into cancer and nutrition cohort. Int J Cancer 2011;129(11):2712–9.
80. de Vrese M, Schrezenmeir J. Probiotics, prebiotics, and synbiotics. Adv Biochem Eng Biotechnol 2008;111:1–66.
81. Arumugam M, Raes J, Pelletier E, et al. Enterotypes of the human gut microbiome. Nature 2011;473(7346):174–80.

82. Corthésy B, Gaskins HR, Mercenier A. Cross-talk between probiotic bacteria and the host immune system. J Nutr 2007;137(3 Suppl 2):781S–90S.
83. Orlando A, Messa C, Linsalata M, et al. Effects of *Lactobacillus rhamnosus* GG on proliferation and polyamine metabolism in HGC-27 human gastric and DLD-1 colonic cancer cell lines. Immunopharmacol Immunotoxicol 2009;31(1):108–16.
84. Lee NK, Park JS, Park E, et al. Adherence and anticarcinogenic effects of *Bacillus polyfermenticus* SCD in the large intestine. Lett Appl Microbiol 2007;44(3): 274–8.
85. Kim Y, Lee D, Kim D, et al. Inhibition of proliferation in colon cancer cell lines and harmful enzyme activity of colon bacteria by *Bifidobacterium adolescentis* SPM0212. Arch Pharm Res 2008;31(4):468–73.
86. Tlaskalová-Hogenová H, Stěpánková R, Kozáková H, et al. The role of gut microbiota (commensal bacteria) and the mucosal barrier in the pathogenesis of inflammatory and autoimmune diseases and cancer: contribution of germ-free and gnotobiotic animal models of human diseases. Cell Mol Immunol 2011; 8(2):110–20.

The Oral Microbiome and Oral Cancer

Laura Wang, MBBS, Ian Ganly, MD, PhD*

KEYWORDS

- Oral microbiome • HOMIM • Oral squamous cell carcinoma • Carcinogenesis

KEY POINTS

- The use of recently developed molecular methods has greatly expanded our knowledge of the composition and function of the oral microbiome in health and disease.
- The oral microbiome differs between normal persons and patients with oral squamous cell carcinoma (OSCC), however no pathognomonic bacterial or bacterial spectrum has yet been identified in OSCC.
- Human responses to the microbiome are not well understood. Prospective studies may help to resolve the temporal order between microbiome changes and the development of oral cancer.
- Research into the oral microbiome holds the key to one day allow for early diagnosis of OSCC and possible ways to modulate the microbiome prophylactically and therapeutically.

INTRODUCTION

Bacteria have been linked to cancer through several mechanisms such as production of toxins, chronic inflammation, and carcinogenic metabolites. Several bacteria are thought to contribute to carcinogenesis in humans. Examples include *Streptococcus bovis* in the pathogenesis of colonic cancer and *Salmonella typhi* in the development of hepatobiliary cancer. None have been more extensively studied than *Helicobacter pylori* and its role in the carcinogenesis of gastric cancer. Collectively, the pathophysiology of bacterial infection leading to cancer may be modeled on the understanding of *H pylori* and gastric cancer. The International Agency for Research on Cancer and the World Health Organization has classified this bacterium as a group 1 human carcinogen. Various pathogenesis pathways have been proposed. Although it is known that *H pylori* produces enzymes that induce gastric mucosal damage, the

Disclosures: None.
Head and Neck Service, Department of Surgery, Memorial Sloan Kettering Cancer Center, 1275 York Avenue, New York, NY 10021, USA
* Corresponding author.
E-mail address: ganlyi@mskcc.org

Clin Lab Med 34 (2014) 711–719
http://dx.doi.org/10.1016/j.cll.2014.08.004
0272-2712/14/$ – see front matter © 2014 Elsevier Inc. All rights reserved.
labmed.theclinics.com

pathogenesis toward gastric cancer largely depends on host immune responses. Individual host genetic polymorphisms determine the physiologic response to infection, altering inflammatory cytokine release, the extent and duration of inflammatory response, and the eventual progression toward cancer. The pathophysiology of *H pylori* infection and eventual disease outcome is a complex interaction between the host and the bacteria, which is further influenced by many yet unidentified environmental variables.

There is increasing evidence that bacteria may have a role in the development of oral cancer. The oral cavity harbors one of the most diverse microbiomes in the human body, including viruses, fungi, protozoa, archaea, and bacteria. The bacterial communities found in the human body are highly complex, with around 1000 species alone in the mouth.[1] The oral microbiome is one of the most complex in the body, second only to that of the colon.[2] Until recently, our understanding of the human microbiome was limited to the 20% to 50% that could be grown in culture media.[1,3,4]

The role that bacteria play in the etiology and predisposition to cancer is of increasing interest, particularly since the development of high-throughput genetic-based assays. With this technology, it has become possible to comprehensively examine entire microbiomes as a functional entity.[5] This review outlines our understanding of the link between the oral microbiome and oral cancer. Although the microbiome includes all organisms of the oral cavity, including viruses, fungi, and archaea, this article focuses on the understanding of bacteria and its association with oral squamous cell carcinoma (OSCC).

METHODS OF BACTERIA DETECTION

Until recently, studies of the human microbiome were based on culture methods, which are highly insensitive because of the large numbers of nonculturable microbes. Over the last decade, the cost of DNA sequencing has dropped exponentially while throughput has increased many-fold. A major advancement has been the adoption of high-throughput, next-generation sequencing methods such as pyrosequencing. 16S rRNA gene pyrosequencing provides an in-depth analysis of microbiomes more cost-effectively than with traditional sequencing techniques. However, this technique is not without its limitations, including inaccuracies and short and partial sequencing reads.[6]

Another commonly used method is a preconstructed microarray developed to detect the most prevalent oral bacterial species. The Human Oral Microbe Identification Microarray (HOMIM) uses specially designed probes to detect 300 to 400 of the most prevalent oral bacterial species including those that have not yet been cultivated,[7] but is limited to previously identified bacterial sequences. Comparisons of pyrosequencing and HOMIM has found them to be highly correlated at the phylum level and highly correlated for common taxa at the genus level. However, pyrosequencing provides a broader spectrum of taxa identification and greater detection sensitivity, and allows for detection of previously undiscovered species.[8]

Metagenomic sequencing is also increasingly cost-effective. Unlike previously described techniques, this method allows for the sequencing of the entire microbiome genome, and offers the advantage of elucidating bacterial phenotype and functional relationships not identified using previous sequencing techniques.[9] Continuing technological developments will enable improved access to accurate, cost-effective hypothesis-testing methods for researchers.

THE NORMAL ORAL FLORA AND PUBLIC DATABASE RESOURCES

Before detecting possible alterations in oral microbiome compositions that are diagnostic or pathogenic of oral cancer, it is necessary to understand the healthy oral microbiome and the differences between individuals and oral cavity subsites. Next-generation sequencing has provided a culture-independent method to comprehensively and accurately document the microbiome in states of health and disease.

Many studies have been dedicated to deciphering the composition of the normal oral microbiome in healthy individuals. These studies reveal that a limited range of bacterial phyla, the most abundant of which are Firmicutes, Bacteroidetes, Proteobacteria, Fusobacteria, and Actinobacteria, inhabit the healthy oral microbiome.[10–14] The most predominant bacterial genus is *Streptococcus* followed by *Prevotella, Veillonella, Neisseria,* and *Haemophilus*.[10,11] It has also been demonstrated that the oral microbiome between individuals differs significantly at the species or strain level.[11,14] Variation also exists within oral cavity sites (ie, lateral vs dorsal tongue, enamel surface, and so forth).[10,11] The oral microbiome remains stable within individuals over time[12,15] and relatively stable across countries.[13]

In the past decade, members of the International Human Microbiome Consortium (IHMC)[16] have prioritized and collaborated on human microbiome research, including the National Institutes of Health (NIH). The NIH initiated the Human Microbiome Project (HMP) with the goals of studying the entire human microbiome and creating a public access reference collection of microbiome sequences.[5] HMP, in conjunction with other members of the IHMC, provides a publicly available human microbiome genome database of sequenced microbes (http://www.hmpdacc.org). Other 16S rRNA gene reference sequences are available from the Ribosomal Database Project[17] (http://rdp.cme.msu.edu) and SILVA[18] (http://www.arb-silva.de). In addition, further classification by taxonomy is available at the Human Oral Microbiome Database[3] (www.homd.org).

ASSOCIATION BETWEEN BACTERIA AND ORAL CANCER
Culture-Based Studies

Poor oral hygiene and periodontal disease has been long been linked with carcinoma of the oral cavity.[19–21] Although there is increasing evidence that the OSCC is associated with changes in the oral microbiome, there is currently no consensus regarding specific changes in the bacterial species. This discord is largely due to the limitation of earlier studies, restricted to the analysis of only a small number of oral bacterial species that can be cultured.[22,23]

Culture-based comparisons of patients with and without OSCC[22–27] indicated bacterial community profiles to be highly correlated at the phylum level but diverse at the genus level. Studies have analyzed bacterial species within tumor lesions and in mucosal bacterial communities superficial to OSCC. In 1997, Nagy and colleagues[22] investigated the biofilms present on the surfaces of OSCC and from adjacent healthy mucosa obtained from 21 patients using culture. The bacterial taxa isolated in increased numbers at tumor sites were *Veillonella, Fusobacterium, Prevotella, Porphyromonas, Actinomyces,* and *Clostridium,* and *Haemophilus, Enterobacteriaceae,* and *Streptococcus* spp. It was concluded that human oral carcinoma surface biofilms harbor significantly increased numbers of both aerobes and anaerobes in comparison with the healthy mucosal surface of the same patient. In another study, Bolz and colleagues[28] described a prospective comparison of surface bacteria in patients with OSCC, high-risk controls, and normal controls. Thirty patients were enlisted in each arm with the aim of identifying characteristic microbiome colonization associated within each group. A culture-based analysis of the 90 swab samples found that the ratio between aerobes and anaerobes was 2:1 in health patients, 1:1 in high-risk patients, and 1:2 in the OSCC group.[28] In 2006, Hooper and colleagues[23] performed an analysis of 20 OSCC samples with corresponding control tissues, with the aim of identifying bacterial species within OSCC tissue. Similarly to Nagy and colleagues, it was seen that some bacteria were uniquely associated with tumor, whereas other species were limited to only normal samples. Examples of bacteria unique to tumor specimens included *Exiguobacterium oxidotolerans*, *Prevotella melaninogenica*, *Staphylococcus aureus*, *Veillonella parvula*, and species of *Micrococcus*.[23]

Streptococcus anginosus DNA sequence was initially found in DNA samples extracted from esophageal cancers. Taking a different approach, several Japanese groups have focused on identification of a single bacterial organism, demonstrating conflicting results regarding the association of *S anginosus* with head and neck cancer (HNC). Tateda and colleagues[25] investigated this association, and found all 68 samples of oral cancer to harbor *S anginosus* on polymerase chain reaction (PCR). Sasaki and colleagues[27] reported similar findings with *S anginosus* DNA detected in 19 of 42 OSCC lesions. Further culture analysis of patient saliva and dental plaque suggested that dental plaque was a likely reservoir of the *S anginosus*.[27] By contrast, when the same Tateda group went on to use improved PCR methods to quantitatively analyze *S anginosus* in OSCC, lesions demonstrated low frequency and small amounts of *S anginosus* DNA in oral cancer tissues. The group acknowledged that *S anginosus* detection methods were not sufficiently reliable for drawing firm conclusions.[26]

Lastly, several studies have detected the presence of *H pylori* in the oral cavity. However, like *S. anginosus*, there is conflicting evidence to support its association with OSCC.[29–32]

Molecular-Based Studies on Bacteria Associated with Oral Cancer

Initial molecular-based studies generally have analyzed limited numbers of bacterial species[33] or have conducted comprehensive analysis on a small sample size.[34–36] Based on these data, one cannot distinguish whether the observed shifts in the microbial community reflect that certain bacteria are more suited to adhere and grow in the cancer microenvironment or whether they are cancer promoting.

Early molecular studies were limited to analysis of a small number of common oral bacteria. In 2005, Mager and colleagues[33] performed a case-match analysis of 45 OSCC and non-OSCC patients to determine the difference in salivary bacterial count. Analysis was limited to 40 common bacteria found in the mouth. Three species, *Capnocytophaga gingivalis*, *P melaninogenica*, and *Streptococcus mitis*, were elevated in the saliva of individuals with OSCC. The group proposed that salivary bacterial counts may be a diagnostic indicator of OSCC.[33]

Pushalkar and colleagues[36] compared the saliva of 3 OSCC patients with that of 2 normal controls. In total, members of 8 phyla of bacteria were detected. Most classified sequences belonged to the phyla Firmicutes (45%) and Bacteroidetes (25%). However, a further 67% of sequences at that time were uncultured bacteria or unclassified groups. In a separate study, the same group went on to investigate the composition of bacteria communities within 10 OSCC samples in comparison with normal tissue resected 5 cm away in the same patient. Samples were processed to include all surface bacteria in addition to bacteria within the tissue. *Streptococcus salivarius*, *Streptococcus gordonii*, *Gemella haemolysans*, *Gemella morbillorum*, *Johnsonella ignava*, and *Streptococcus parasanguinis* I were highly associated with tumor site, whereas *Granulicatella adiacens* was prevalent at the nontumor site. *Streptococcus intermedius* was present in 70% of both nontumor and tumor sites.[37]

A similar investigation of bacterial composition of 10 OSCC tissue samples in comparison with normal adjacent tissue was performed by Hooper and colleagues[35] in 2007. In contrast to Pushalkar and colleagues, this group removed all surface bacteria from tissue samples through betadine immersion, limiting analysis to only bacteria within tissues. Although no statistically significant differences in bacterial composition were found, several trends were noted. Tumor groups harbored more *Clavibacter michiganensis*, *Fusobacterium naviforme*, and *Ralstonia insidiosa* compared with control samples from adjacent tissue. By contrast, control samples demonstrated isolates of *G adiacens*, *Porphyromonas gingivalis*, *Sphingomonas* sp PC5.28, and *Streptococcus mitis/oralis*.

More recently, Schmidt and colleagues[14] looked at mucosal bacteria communities of 13 patients with OSCC or precancers in addition to normal individuals. To account for interindividual differences seen in the oral microbiome, samples were obtained from the contralateral tongue as control samples (ie, each patient was his or her own control). When comparing microbiome composition of the ipsilateral lesion and the contralateral control mucosa, it was seen that in OSCC and precancer patients the microbiome over the tumor had a significant reduction in the abundance of Firmicutes represented by *Streptococcus* and Actinobacteria represented by *Rothia*, and an increase in the abundance of Fusobacteria represented by *Fusobacterium* when compared with the normal contralateral sample, a difference that is not present in noncancer patients. When comparing the overall microbiomes of individuals with OSCC or precancer with that of individuals with no such lesions, OSCC and precancer patients had a greater abundance of Bacteroidetes including several *Prevotella* species, for example, *Prevotella intermedia* and *P melaninogenica*, in addition to unclassified species.

POSSIBLE MECHANISMS OF CARCINOGENESIS
Interplay with Alcohol and Smoking

The pathogenesis of OSCC is mainly attributed to the effects of smoking and heavy alcohol consumption. However, other modifying risk factors including infection with *Candida* species,[22] virus,[38] and poor oral cavity hygiene[39] have been identified. The strongest epidemiologic and etiologic link between oral microbial infection and oral cancer is perhaps through the bacterial conversion of ethanol to acetaldehyde (ALD), a recognized carcinogen. Other likely links between oral bacteria and cancer promotion include the generation of other carcinogenic substances, such as nitrosamine,[40] through chronic inflammation,[41] and the direct effects of bacterial toxins on cell signaling.[42]

Alcohol

Alcohol itself is not known to be carcinogenic. However, ALD, its first metabolite, may produce genetic aberrations. In 1997, Homann and colleagues[43] performed an in vivo study from the saliva of 10 healthy volunteers before and after a chlorhexidine mouthwash treatment regime. Mouthwash was found to lead to both a reduction in bacteria and a 50% decrease in ALD after alcohol intake. Of interest, it was noted that volunteers with gram-positive aerobic bacteria and yeasts were associated with higher ALD production.

The same group later went on to evaluate the role of dental status on the microbial production of ALD from alcohol in the saliva samples of 132 volunteers. The in vitro salivary ALD production was then related to the dental scores after adjusting for variables including smoking and alcohol consumption. Poor dental status was shown to lead to a 2-fold increase in salivary ALD production from ethanol. These results highlight the role of oral bacteria in the risk of oral cancer associated with ethanol drinking.[44]

Kurkivuori and colleagues[45] showed that viridans-group streptococci may play a role in metabolizing ethanol to ALD in the mouth. Sixteen different strains of viridans-group streptococci were incubated with ethanol and measured for level of ALD production. In particular, strains of S salivarius, S intermedius, and S mitis produced high amounts of ALD with corresponding significant alcohol dehydrogenase (ADH)-enzyme activity.

In a study of more than 400 HNC patients and 500 controls, Tsai and colleagues[46] investigated the interplay between alcohol consumption, oral hygiene, and genetics polymorphisms of the alcohol-metabolizing genes ADH1b and ALDH2. This study is the first to show that the association between alcohol drinking and HNC risk may be modified by oral hygiene based on genetic polymorphisms. The investigators concluded that in addition to promoting abstinence or reduction of alcohol drinking to decrease the occurrence of HNC, improving oral hygiene practices may also provide benefit.

Smoking

Studies have demonstrated that smoking affects the composition of the bacterial communities in the oral cavity, including the salivary microbiome of healthy smokers and nonsmokers.[34,47] In addition, in vitro studies have shown that bacteria may play a role in increased activation of carcinogenic nitrosamines.[40] The mechanisms linking bacterial activity to propagation of carcinogenesis through smoking have not been well elucidated, and definitive clinical studies are lacking.

Other Mechanisms of Bacterial Carcinogenesis

The cellular mechanism of DNA damage by H pylori is well understood,[42] but those for oral bacteria are less well studied. The bacterial species associated with cancer etiology are diverse. However, common characteristics can be observed. As seen with H pylori, S typhi, and S bovis infections, typically years or even decades pass between acquiring the infection and cancer development. The chronic exposure to the infective bacteria leads the host immune system, producing typical features of chronic inflammation that can lead to DNA damage. It has also been proposed that some bacteria can produce toxins that disrupt cellular signaling, leading to the disruption of normal cell regulation, while others can produce toxins that directly damage DNA.[42,48] Others have hypothesized that microbial populations contribute to oral cancer through aberrant DNA methylation of cancer-associated genes and other epigenetic modifications in inflammation.[34]

SUMMARY

Next-generation sequencing methods have undoubtedly advanced human microbiome research. The use of recently developed molecular methods has greatly expanded our knowledge of the composition and function of the oral microbiome in health and disease. This area of research is supported through well-structured collaborations internationally and nationally, resulting in publicly available reference sequencing for human microbiomes and preconstructed microarray panels available for standardized research approaches.

Despite increasing technology and interest in the relationships between the oral microbiome and the development of oral cancer, much remains to be done. Although it is apparent that the oral microbiome differs between normal and OSCC patients, no pathognomonic bacterial or bacterial spectrum has yet been identified in OSCC.

Variations in human responses to the microbiome are not well understood. The issue of reverse causation also needs to be addressed in future research studies. Prospective studies may help to resolve the temporal order between microbiome changes and the development of oral cancer. Research of the oral microbiome holds the key to one day allow for early diagnosis of OSCC, and possible ways to modulate the microbiome prophylactically and therapeutically.

REFERENCES

1. Dewhirst F, Chen T, Izard J, et al. The human oral microbiome. J Bacteriol 2010; 192:5002–17. http://dx.doi.org/10.1128/JB.00542-10.
2. Huttenhower C, Gevers D, Knight R, et al. Structure, function and diversity of the healthy human microbiome. Nature 2012;486:207–14. http://dx.doi.org/10.1038/nature11234.
3. Chen T, Yu W, Izard J, et al. The Human Oral Microbiome Database: a web accessible resource for investigating oral microbe taxonomic and genomic information. Database (Oxford) 2010;2010:baq013. http://dx.doi.org/10.1093/database/baq013.
4. Wade W. Non-culturable bacteria in complex commensal populations. Adv Appl Microbiol 2004;54:93–106.
5. Peterson J, Garges S, Giovanni M, et al. The NIH Human Microbiome Project. Genome Res 2009;19:2317–23. http://dx.doi.org/10.1101/gr.096651.109.
6. Ahn J, Chen C, Hayes R. Oral microbiome and oral and gastrointestinal cancer risk. Cancer Causes Control 2012;23:399–404. http://dx.doi.org/10.1007/s10552-011-9892-7.
7. Abboud B, Sleilaty G, Braidy C, et al. Careful examination of thyroid specimen intraoperatively to reduce incidence of inadvertent parathyroidectomy during thyroid surgery. Arch Otolaryngol Head Neck Surg 2007;133:1105–10.
8. Ahn J, Yang L, Paster B, et al. Oral microbiome profiles: 16S rRNA pyrosequencing and microarray assay comparison. PLoS One 2011;6:e22788. http://dx.doi.org/10.1371/journal.pone.0022788.
9. Sharpton T. An introduction to the analysis of shotgun metagenomic data. Front Plant Sci 2014;5:209. http://dx.doi.org/10.3389/fpls.2014.00209.
10. Aas J, Paster B, Stokes L, et al. Defining the normal bacterial flora of the oral cavity. J Clin Microbiol 2005;43:5721–32.
11. Bik E, Long C, Armitage G, et al. Bacterial diversity in the oral cavity of 10 healthy individuals. ISME J 2010;4:962–74. http://dx.doi.org/10.1038/ismej.2010.30.
12. Lazarevic V, Whiteson K, Hernandez D, et al. Study of inter- and intra-individual variations in the salivary microbiota. BMC Genomics 2010;11:523. http://dx.doi.org/10.1186/471-2164-11-523.
13. Nasidze I, Li J, Quinque D, et al. Global diversity in the human salivary microbiome. Genome Res 2009;19:636–43. http://dx.doi.org/10.1101/gr.084616.108.
14. Schmidt B, Kuczynski J, Bhattacharya A, et al. Changes in abundance of oral microbiota associated with oral cancer. PLoS One 2014;9:e98741. http://dx.doi.org/10.1371/journal.pone.0098741.
15. Costello E, Lauber C, Hamady M, et al. Bacterial community variation in human body habitats across space and time. Science 2009;326:1694–7. http://dx.doi.org/10.126/science.1177486.
16. International Human Microbiome Consortium. Available at: http://www.human-microbiome.org. Accessed July 15, 2014.

17. Cole J, Wang Q, Cardenas E, et al. The Ribosomal Database Project: improved alignments and new tools for rRNA analysis. Nucleic Acids Res 2009;37: D141–5. http://dx.doi.org/10.1093/nar/gkn879.

18. Quast C, Pruesse E, Yilmaz P, et al. The SILVA ribosomal RNA gene database project: improved data processing and web-based tools. Nucleic Acids Res 2013;41:D590–6. http://dx.doi.org/10.1093/nar/gks219.

19. Spitz M. Epidemiology and risk factors for head and neck cancer. Semin Oncol 1994;21:281–8.

20. Velly A, Franco E, Schlecht N, et al. Relationship between dental factors and risk of upper aerodigestive tract cancer. Oral Oncol 1998;34:284–91.

21. Tezal M, Sullivan M, Reid M, et al. Chronic periodontitis and the risk of tongue cancer. Arch Otolaryngol Head Neck Surg 2007;133:450–4.

22. Nagy K, Sonkodi I, Szoke I, et al. The microflora associated with human oral carcinomas. Oral Oncol 1998;34:304–8.

23. Hooper S, Crean S, Lewis M, et al. Viable bacteria present within oral squamous cell carcinoma tissue. J Clin Microbiol 2006;44:1719–25.

24. Nagy K, Szoke I, Sonkodi I, et al. Inhibition of microflora associated with oral malignancy. Oral Oncol 2000;36:32–6.

25. Tateda M, Shiga K, Saijo S, et al. *Streptococcus anginosus* in head and neck squamous cell carcinoma: implication in carcinogenesis. Int J Mol Med 2000;6: 699–703.

26. Morita E, Narikiyo M, Yano A, et al. Different frequencies of *Streptococcus anginosus* infection in oral cancer and esophageal cancer. Cancer Sci 2003;94: 492–6.

27. Sasaki M, Yamaura C, Ohara-Nemoto Y, et al. *Streptococcus anginosus* infection in oral cancer and its infection route. Oral Dis 2005;11:151–6.

28. Bolz J, Dosa E, Schubert J, et al. Bacterial colonization of microbial biofilms in oral squamous cell carcinoma. Clin Oral Investig 2014;18:409–14. http://dx.doi.org/10.1007/s00784-013-1007-2.

29. Fernando N, Jayakumar G, Perera N, et al. Presence of *Helicobacter pylori* in betel chewers and non betel chewers with and without oral cancers. BMC Oral Health 2009;9:23. http://dx.doi.org/10.1186/472-6831-9-23.

30. Dayama A, Srivastava V, Shukla M, et al. *Helicobacter pylori* and oral cancer: possible association in a preliminary case control study. Asian Pac J Cancer Prev 2011;12:1333–6.

31. Singh K, Kumar S, Jaiswal M, et al. Absence of *Helicobacter pylori* in oral mucosal lesions. J Indian Med Assoc 1998;96:177–8.

32. Okuda K, Ishihara K, Miura T, et al. *Helicobacter pylori* may have only a transient presence in the oral cavity and on the surface of oral cancer. Microbiol Immunol 2000;44:385–8.

33. Mager D, Haffajee A, Devlin P, et al. The salivary microbiota as a diagnostic indicator of oral cancer: a descriptive, non-randomized study of cancer-free and oral squamous cell carcinoma subjects. J Transl Med 2005;3:27.

34. Bebek G, Bennett K, Funchain P, et al. Microbiomic subprofiles and MDR1 promoter methylation in head and neck squamous cell carcinoma. Hum Mol Genet 2012;21:1557–65. http://dx.doi.org/10.093/hmg/ddr593.

35. Hooper S, Crean S, Fardy M, et al. A molecular analysis of the bacteria present within oral squamous cell carcinoma. J Med Microbiol 2007;56:1651–9.

36. Pushalkar S, Mane S, Ji X, et al. Microbial diversity in saliva of oral squamous cell carcinoma. FEMS Immunol Med Microbiol 2011;61:269–77. http://dx.doi.org/10.1111/j.574-695X.2010.00773.x.

37. Pushalkar S, Ji X, Li Y, et al. Comparison of oral microbiota in tumor and non-tumor tissues of patients with oral squamous cell carcinoma. BMC Microbiol 2012;12:144. http://dx.doi.org/10.1186/471-2180-12-144.

38. Kobayashi I, Shima K, Saito I, et al. Prevalence of Epstein-Barr virus in oral squamous cell carcinoma. J Pathol 1999;189:34–9.

39. Tezal M, Sullivan M, Hyland A, et al. Chronic periodontitis and the incidence of head and neck squamous cell carcinoma. Cancer Epidemiol Biomarkers Prev 2009;18:2406–12. http://dx.doi.org/10.1158/055-9965.EPI-09-0334.

40. Verna L, Whysner J, Williams G. N-nitrosodiethylamine mechanistic data and risk assessment: bioactivation, DNA-adduct formation, mutagenicity, and tumor initiation. Pharmacol Ther 1996;71:57–81.

41. Meurman J. Oral microbiota and cancer. J Oral Microbiol 2010;2. http://dx.doi.org/10.3402/jom.v2i0.5195.

42. Lax A. Opinion: bacterial toxins and cancer–a case to answer? Nat Rev Microbiol 2005;3:343–9.

43. Homann N, Jousimies-Somer H, Jokelainen K, et al. High acetaldehyde levels in saliva after ethanol consumption: methodological aspects and pathogenetic implications. Carcinogenesis 1997;18:1739–43.

44. Homann N, Tillonen J, Rintamaki H, et al. Poor dental status increases acetaldehyde production from ethanol in saliva: a possible link to increased oral cancer risk among heavy drinkers. Oral Oncol 2001;37:153–8.

45. Kurkivuori J, Salaspuro V, Kaihovaara P, et al. Acetaldehyde production from ethanol by oral streptococci. Oral Oncol 2007;43:181–6.

46. Tsai S, Wong T, Ou C, et al. The interplay between alcohol consumption, oral hygiene, ALDH2 and ADH1B in the risk of head and neck cancer. Int J Cancer 2014; 10:28885.

47. Chen J, Bittinger K, Charlson E, et al. Associating microbiome composition with environmental covariates using generalized UniFrac distances. Bioinformatics 2012;28:2106–13. http://dx.doi.org/10.1093/bioinformatics/bts342.

48. Lax A. The *Pasteurella multocida* toxin: a new paradigm for the link between bacterial infection and cancer. Curr Top Microbiol Immunol 2012;361:131–44. http://dx.doi.org/10.1007/82_2012_236.

Microbiome, Innate Immunity, and Esophageal Adenocarcinoma

Jonathan Baghdadi, MD[a], Noami Chaudhary, MD[a],
Zhiheng Pei, MD, PhD[a,b,c], Liying Yang, MD[a,*]

KEYWORDS

- Reflux • Barrett esophagus • Adenocarcinoma • Microbiome
- Chronic inflammation • Viruses • Bacteria • Innate immunity

KEY POINTS

- With the development of culture-independent technique, a complex microbiome has been established and described in the distal esophagus.
- Over recent decades, the incidence of esophageal adenocarcinoma (EAC), a relatively rare cancer with high mortality, has increased dramatically in the United States.
- Several studies documenting an altered microbiome associated with EAC and its precedents (ie, Barrett esophagus and reflux esophagitis) suggest that dysbiosis may be contributing to carcinogenesis, potentially mediated by interactions with toll-like receptors.
- Investigations attempting to associate viruses, in particular human papilloma virus, with EAC have not been as consistent. Regardless, currently available data are cross-sectional and therefore cannot prove causal relationships.
- Prospectively, microbiome studies open a new avenue to the understanding of the etiology and pathogenesis of reflux disorders and EAC.

INTRODUCTION

Esophageal adenocarcinoma (EAC) is a relatively rare but aggressive cancer that has been increasing in incidence, particularly among white men.[1-3] EAC typically develops in the distal esophagus in response to mucosal injury, such as with exposure to gastric

This work was supported in part by grants R03CA159414, R01CA159036, R01AI110372, R21ES023421, U01CA18237, and UH3CA140233 from the National Cancer Institute at the National Institutes of Health Human Microbiome Project and by the Department of Veterans Affairs, Veterans Health Administration, Office of Research.

[a] Department of Medicine, New York University School of Medicine, 550 1st Avenue, New York, NY 10016, USA; [b] Department of Veterans Affairs New York Harbor Healthcare System, 423 East 23rd street, New York, NY 10010, USA; [c] Department of Pathology, New York University School of Medicine, 550 1st Avenue, New York, NY 10016, USA
* Corresponding author. New York University School of Medicine, 550 1st Avenue, New York, NY 10016.
E-mail address: liying.yang@nyumc.org

reflux, and is preceded by Barrett esophagus (BE), a form of epithelial metaplasia. Beyond demographics, the major risk factors for EAC are gastroesophageal reflux disease (GERD), cigarette smoking, obesity, and low fruit and vegetable consumption. At a single cancer center, these risk factors represented a combined population-attributable risk of nearly 80%.[4]

The relationship between GERD and EAC is complex. Symptomatic GERD is a strong risk factor for EAC,[5,6] with increasing odds of an association as symptoms manifest for a longer duration or with increased frequency.[7] However, esophagitis may develop in patients without significant acid exposure.[8] The complications of GERD (esophagitis,[9] BE,[10] and EAC[4]) likewise may arise in the absence of preceding symptoms. Thus, acid reflux alone may not fully account for the pathogenesis of EAC. We hypothesize that characteristics of the esophageal microbiome facilitate the development of disease.

MICROBIOME OF THE NORMAL ESOPHAGUS

Early work to characterize an esophageal microbiome was undertaken by surgeons in the hope of preventing infections after thoracotomy.[11–14] These studies used conventional bacterial culture and therefore missed most of the indigenous esophageal biota, which is in a viable but nonculturable state.[15,16] More recent approaches to characterize complex microbial communities have used polymerase chain reaction (PCR) of 16S ribosomal RNA[17] to better characterize nonculturable bacteria.

Using culture-independent technique to examine biopsies of normal esophagus, Pei and colleagues[18] first described a complex bacterial biota in the distal esophagus. Ninety-five species were identified, including members of 6 phyla: Firmicutes, Bacteroides, Actinobacteria, Proteobacteria, Fusobacteria, and TM7. Two phyla seen in the oral cavity, Spirochaetes and Deferribacteres, were not present. Remarkably, findings were similar across specimens, suggesting a stable esophageal biota that is distinct from the flora of the oropharynx, stomach, or food bolus in transit. Microscopic examination of the tissue confirmed a close association of the bacteria with the cell surfaces of the mucosal epithelium in situ, suggesting a residential, rather than a transient, biota.

MICROBIOME IN DISEASE STATES

In 2005, Pei and colleagues[19] undertook the first study to apply cultivation-independent technique to the microbiome in esophageal disease, with the goal of demonstrating feasibility. Two 16S rRNA gene clones were recovered and examined from each of the esophageal biopsies taken from 24 subjects (9 with normal mucosa, 12 with GERD, and 3 with BE). As expected, bacterial signals were successfully detected in all biopsies, and the overall diversity and community membership resembled those of the normal esophageal microbiome.

A more comprehensive approach was taken by Yang and colleagues[20] in 2009. Representing one of the largest human microbiome studies to date, a total of 6800 16S rRNA gene clones from 34 subjects were analyzed by Sanger sequencing. Using both unsupervised and phenotype-guided clustering analyses, samples were found to contain 1 of 2 distinct microbiomes. Microbiome type I was mainly associated with normal esophagus and was predominated by gram-positive bacteria from the Firmicutes phylum, of which *Streptococcus* was the most dominant genus. Microbiome type II had greater proportion of gram-negative anaerobes/microaerophiles (phyla Bacteroidetes, Proteobacteria, Fusobacteria, and Spirochaetes) and primarily correlated with reflux esophagitis (RE) (odds ratio, 15.4) and BE (odds ratio, 16.5). The microbiome did not differ between patients with GERD and patients with BE.

In a subsequent study from Japan, Liu and colleagues[21] compared the bacterial populations present in biopsies taken from 18 Japanese subjects (6 each with normal esophagus, RE, and BE). A unique test performed was quantification of total bacterial loads by 16S rRNA PCR. Notably, approximately 10^6 to 10^7 colony-forming units were counted in each sample, irrespective of disease. This finding suggests that changes in the relative abundance of taxa, rather than differences in absolute bacterial loads, are likely more relevant to esophageal diseases. Although far from comprehensive (only approximately 24 clones were sequenced per sample), *Veillonella* (19%), *Prevotella* (12%), *Neisseria* (4%), and *Fusobacterium* (9%) were found to be prevalent in patients with RE and BE but were not detected in controls. These observations support the earlier work of Pei and colleagues[19] and Yang and colleagues,[20] confirming that the esophageal microbiome is reliably altered in reflux disorders (**Fig. 1**).

Historical milestones		**Studies on esophageal microbial community**
		CULTURE/CULTURE-INDEPENDENT
Microscopic single-celled organisms Leeuwenhoek AV	**1676**	
Germ theory of disease Pasteur L	**1862**	
Koch's postulates Koch R	**1882**	
DNA Sequencing Sanger F	**1977**	
16S rRNA sequences for taxonomy Woese C	**1977**	
	1981	Bacteria were cultured from 64% aspirates of esophageal cancer (n = 79) (14 species). Lau WF
	1982	Bacteria were cultured from all 12 biopsies of esophageal cancer (15 species). Finlay IG
	1983	Bacteria were cultured from all 101 aspirates of esophageal cancer (32 species). Mannell A
Identification of bacterial cause for human diseases by culture-independent method Relman DA	**1990**	
Sequencing whole bacterial genome TIGR	**1995**	
	1998	Bacteria were cultured from 67% aspirates of normal esophagus (n = 30) (11 species). Gagliardi D
	2004	Bacteria were identified by culture-independent method in all 4 biopsies of normal esophagus (95 species). Pei Z
	2004	Bacteria were identified by culture-independent method in 87% biopsies of normal esophagus (n = 20) (7 species). Narikiyo M
	2005	Bacteria were identified by culture-independent method in all 24 biopsies of esophagitis and Barrett esophagus (39 species). Pei Z
High-throughput pyrosequencing 454 Life Science	**2006**	
	2007	Bacteria were cultured from 50%-71% biopsies/aspirates of normal and Barrett esophagus (n = 14) (46 species). Macfarlane Z
Human Microbiome project NIH	**2007**	
	2009	Bacteria were identified by culture-independent method in all 34 biopsies of normal esophagus, esophagitis and Barrett's esophagus (166 species). Yang L
	2013	Bacteria were identified by culture-independent method in all 18 biopsies/aspirates of reflux esophagitis and Barrett esophagus (number of species not reported). Liu N
	2013	Bacteria were cultured from all 151 biopsies of normal esophagus, GERD, Barrett esophagus, and cancer (111 species). Blackett KL

Fig. 1. Timeline of esophageal microbiology.

INFLUENCE OF TOLL-LIKE RECEPTORS

Toll-like receptors (TLRs) expressed in the microenvironment of the esophageal mucosa mediate the interaction of the immune system with the microbiome. TLRs coordinate between a state of homeostasis and a state of injury.[22] Thus, TLRs have become an area of interest as potential mediators of inflammation-related carcinogenesis.[23] In particular, TLR3, TLR4, TLR5, and TLR9 have been suggested as potential mediators of the progression from reflux disorders to EAC (**Table 1**).

Toll-like Receptor 3 and Toll-like Receptor 4

TLR3[24] and TLR4[25] have been implicated in GERD-spectrum disorders largely by documentation of their expression and expression of their downstream products (cyclooxygenase-2 [COX-2], interleukin-8 [IL-8], nuclear factor-κB [NF-κB], and nitric oxide [NO]) in tissue samples and ex vivo cell culture.[26–32] In a murine model, inhibition of COX-2 reduced progression of BE to EAC.[33] In biopsies of RE, higher levels of IL-8 are associated with dysplasia and EAC,[34,35] as well as recurrence of symptoms after cessation of acid-reducing therapy.[36] NF-κB is considered a promoter of inflammation-associated carcinogenesis[37] and mediates the initial metaplastic changes that lead to BE.[38] Blockade of NF-κB activity has been shown to reduce the acid-induced inflammatory response in cell lines derived from EAC.[39] In mice, TLR4-mediated release of NO by colon cancer cells treated with lipopolysaccharide (LPS) has been shown to suppress cytotoxic T-cell and natural killer cell activity, promoting tumor growth and shortening mouse survival.[40] NO release has been suggested as an explanation for LPS-induced dysfunction of the lower esophageal sphincter.[41]

Thus, a body of evidence is mounting to suggest a role for TLR3 and TLR4 in the pathogenesis of EAC. One of the exogenous ligands for TLR4 is LPS, a component of the cell membrane of gram-negative bacteria.[42] Based on the findings of Yang and colleagues,[20] it can be proposed that a shift in the esophageal microbiome in GERD-spectrum disorders toward a predominance of gram-negative bacteria might preferentially stimulate TLR4, triggering a larger and more carcinogenic inflammatory cascade.

Unfortunately, the in situ ligand for TLR3 remains unidentified, making a plausible biological pathway difficult to hypothesize. The natural ligand for TLR3 is viral double-stranded DNA, but no virus, with the possible exception of human papilloma virus (HPV), has been identified as playing a consistent role in GERD-spectrum disorders.

Toll-like Receptor 5 and Toll-like Receptor 9

Less evidence is available to support roles for TLR5 or TLR9 in the development of EAC. In a case series from a single medical center, TLR5 expression within the esophageal epithelium was shown to increase in a stepwise manner with progression from normal to dysplastic and eventually neoplastic states.[43] Meanwhile, TLR9, when strongly expressed by EAC, has been associated with markers of poor prognosis (advanced stage, high-grade pathology, tumor unresectability, lymph node involvement, and distant metastases), as well as shortened survival.[44]

Therefore, more research will need to be performed before a plausible role in for TLR5 and TLR9 in the pathogenic sequence can be hypothesized. The ligands for TLR5 and TLR9 are bacterial flagellin[45] and bacterial DNA,[46] respectively. Thus, although the esophageal microbiome likely plays a role in their activation, it is unclear how the altered microbiome documented by Yang and colleagues[20] might interact with TLR5 and TLR9 differently from the normal one.

Table 1
Summary of studies linking TLRs to GERD, BE, and EAC

Category	TLR3	TLR4	TLR5	TLR9
Function	Intracellular. Recognizes viral dsRNA and induces the activation of NF-κB and production of Type 1 interferons.	Cell surface. Implicated in signal transduction events induced by LPS found in most gram-negative bacteria.	Cell surface. Protein product recognizes bacterial flagellin. Activation of this receptor mobilizes NF-κB.	Intracellular. Recognizes unmethylated CpG sequences in DNA molecules.
Disease	Esophagitis, GERD	BE	BE, EAC	EAC
Specimen	Biopsy	Biopsy	Biopsy	Biopsy
Results	Increased TLR3 expression on EAC-derived epithelial cell lines (HET-1A, TE-1, and TE-7). TLR2+ immune cells but not TLR2 expression, were seen in biopsies from patients with both GERD and eosinophilic esophagitis.	NF-κB activation on TLR4 stimulation. Increased IL-8 expression and activation on TLR4 activation. Increased COX-2 expression in BE on TLR4 activation.	TLR5 overexpression was a sensitive and specific marker in identification of dysplastic lesions in BE. Dysplastic lesions and adenocarcinomas showed increased TLR5 expression. TLR5 had no prognostic value in EAC.	TLR9 was expressed in all EAC tumors. High TLR9 expression correlated with advanced tumor stage, tumor unresectability, poor differentiation, and high proliferation. Cumulative 10-year survival for patients with EAC with weak TLR9 expression was 35.2% and 9.3%, respectively, for patients with strong TLR9 expression.
Reference	24	25	43	44

Abbreviations: BE, Barrett esophagus; COX, cyclo-oxygenase; EAC, esophageal adenocarcinoma; GERD, gastroesophageal reflux disease; IL, interleukin; LPS, lipopolysaccharide; NF-κB, nuclear factor κB; TLR, Toll-like receptor.
Data from Refs.[24,25,43,44]

ROLES OF VIRUSES

HPV is the subject of interest as a potential driver of tumorigenesis in the distal esophagus. HPV is known to have a strong association with esophageal squamous cell carcinoma,[47] but its role in the development of EAC is much less clear. Outside of the esophagus, HPV has an established role in the development of cancers of the cervix[48] and oropharynx.[49] Analogies have been drawn between the pathogenesis of cervical cancer and EAC,[50] based in part on similar premalignant changes in the epithelial cell expression of human leukocyte antigen (HLA) that are suspected to affect the immune response to HPV.[51] However, investigations attempting to document HPV in EAC and its premalignant conditions have yielded mixed results.[52]

In the largest study to address this topic, Rajendra and colleagues[53] evaluated biopsies from 261 Australian patients by PCR for HPV DNA. HPV, when identified, was evaluated for transcriptional activity by quantification of oncogene mRNA expression and protein immunohistochemistry. Twenty-four (68.6%) of 35 patients with dysplastic BE and 18 (66.7%) of 27 with EAC were found to be HPV-positive, compared with 17 (22.1%) of 77 patients with nondysplastic BE and 22 (18.0%) of 122 controls. Most HPV strains detected were high-risk subtypes (16 and 18), with markers for transcriptional activity found predominantly in dysplastic and malignant samples. Although the investigators noted that the background prevalence of oral HPV is higher in Australians[54] than Americans,[55] these data support a potential role for HPV in the pathway from metaplasia to dysplasia and neoplasia in the esophagus.

The only other study to show a robust association between BE and HPV is a biopsy series from Mexico.[56] HPV was detected in 27 (96%) of 28 biopsies of BE, compared with only 6 (26%) of 23 samples with esophagitis. However, samples were not stratified by dysplasia, and no controls were available for comparison. Regardless, these data seem to suggest that HPV is, at the very least, not uncommon in the setting of distal esophageal metaplasia.

Other studies have failed to show a similar connection. In an American biopsy series,[57] HPV DNA was detected in 23 (27.4%) of 84 cases of BE, 11 (31%) of 36 cases of EAC, and in 7 (24%) of 29 healthy controls. No statistical differences were found between groups with regard to the presence of HPV, the presence of high-risk versus low-risk subtypes, or immunohistochemistry for P16INK4a (a viral product that is used as a marker for activity of infection). However, only 6 of the cases of BE evaluated were dysplastic, which may explain the different findings in this study when compared with those of Rajendra[53] (**Table 2**).[58]

Still more investigations from America have shown HPV to be entirely absent from biopsies of nondysplastic BE[59] or frozen surgical specimens from resected EAC. In a study from the United Kingdom, HPV was identified in only 1 of 73 biopsies of BE.[60] In an Italian biopsy series, HPV DNA was detected in 2 (10%) of 20 cases of EAC, compared with 8 (30%) of 27 cases of RE.[61] These results are difficult to reconcile with those of Acevedo-Nuno and colleagues[56] and suggest that HPV is not common in EAC and its precursors. Although background geographic variation in prevalence of HPV may explain these disparities, the low frequency of HPV in American studies stands in stark contrast to the rising incidence of EAC over recent decades in the United States.

Regarding other viruses, a study evaluating surgical frozen sections by PCR for adenovirus, cytomegalovirus, and Epstein-Barr virus failed to show any differences between patients with EAC and controls.[62]

Table 2
A summary of previous studies that examined HPV infection in BE or EAC

Study First Author, Year	Region	Cases n (BE/EAC)	Case Tissue Examined (Design)	Control Subjects n	Control Tissue Examined	Method of HPV Testing	% HPV Positive
Acevedo-Nuno et al,[56] 2004	Mexico	45 (28/17)	Lesion-targeted biopsy	23 esophagitis	Gastroesophageal junction	PCR	96% BE, 26% controls (P<.01).
						IHC	Increasing correlation with esophagitis, BE, and EAC (P = .000)
Rai et al,[60] 2008	United Kingdom	73 (73/0)	Biopsy from suspected BE lesion	None	N/A	PCR	1.4% in BE
Wang et al,[52] 2010	United States	34 (0/34)	Tumor site	54 ESCC biopsies	Tumor site	PCR	52.9% in EAC vs 66.7% in ESCC (P = .2)
Iyer et al,[57] 2011	North America	116 (80/36)	Lesion-targeted biopsy	29 normal biopsies	Biopsy at gastroesophageal junction	PCR	28% BE, 31% EAC, 21% control

Abbreviations: BE, Barrett esophagus; EAC, esophageal adenocarcinoma; ESCC, esophageal squamous cell carcinoma; HPV, human papillomavirus; IHC, immunohistochemistry; N/A, not applicable; PCR, polymerase chain reaction.

From El-Serag HB, Hollier JM, Gravitt P, et al. Human papillomavirus and the risk of Barrett's esophagus. Dis Esophagus 2013;26:520; with permission.

Helicobacter pylori

Meta-analyses and cross-sectional evaluation of biopsies have shown an inverse relationship between the presence of *H pylori* and GERD-spectrum disorders.[63–65] However, eradication of *H pylori* does not induce new cases of GERD, nor does it worsen GERD symptoms (except in patients with hiatal hernia and corpus gastritis).[66] The role of *H pylori* in the pathogenesis of GERD, BE, and EAC remains an unclear and controversial topic that has been extensively reviewed elsewhere.[67]

POTENTIAL ROLE OF THE MICROBIOME IN DISEASE

Although the microbiome has been implicated in inflammation and carcinogenesis elsewhere in the gastrointestinal tract,[68] studies to date of the distal esophagus have been cross-sectional and therefore unable to establish a causal relationship. Given that the gut microbiome has been shown to be heritable,[69] it is unclear whether the variant microbiome demonstrated by Yang and colleagues[20] was acquired in response to environmental factors, such as antibiotics,[70] was deposited directly by gastric reflux, or is stable from childhood. Likewise, it cannot be determined whether this variant microbiome caused disease by induction of abnormal lower esophageal sphincter function, accelerated disease by potentiating inflammation via interaction with TLRs, predisposed toward disease by altering the immune response to incipient cancer, or resulted from changes in the local microenvironment related to acid exposure. Longitudinal studies will be necessary to parse out temporal relationships.

PERSPECTIVES

Esophageal microbiology is an understudied field, especially in EAC. Prospective studies to explore whether the microbiome changes before or after onset of disease are the next logical step to evaluate causality. A large-scale study on this topic has been funded under the National Institutes of Health Human Microbiome Project and may fill the knowledge gap. Large cohorts, such as the National Cancer Institute–Prostate, Lung, Colorectal, and Ovarian Cancer Screening Trial Cohort and the American Cancer Society Cancer Prevention Study II Cohort, have access to tissue samples collected before cancer diagnosis and therefore should prove invaluable to further characterize the role of the esophageal microbiome in carcinogenesis.[71]

REFERENCES

1. Devesa SS, Blot WJ, Fraumeni JF Jr. Changing patterns in the incidence of esophageal and gastric carcinoma in the United States. Cancer 1998;83: 2049–53.
2. Daly JM, Karnell LH, Menck HR. National cancer data base report on esophageal carcinoma. Cancer 1996;78:1820–8.
3. Brown LM, Devesa SS, Chow WH. Incidence of adenocarcinoma of the esophagus among white Americans by sex, stage, and age. J Natl Cancer Inst 2008; 100:1184–7.
4. Engel LS, Chow WH, Vaughan TL, et al. Population attributable risks of esophageal and gastric cancers. J Natl Cancer Inst 2003;95:1404–13.
5. Lagergren J, Bergstrom R, Lindgren A, et al. Symptomatic gastroesophageal reflux as a risk factor for esophageal adenocarcinoma. N Engl J Med 1999; 340:825–31.

6. Rubenstein JH, Taylor JB. Meta-analysis: the association of oesophageal adenocarcinoma with symptoms of gastro-oesophageal reflux. Aliment Pharmacol Ther 2010;32:1222–7.

7. Farrow DC, Vaughan TL, Sweeney C, et al. Gastroesophageal reflux disease, use of H-2 receptor antagonists, and risk of esophageal and gastric cancer. Cancer Causes Control 2000;11:231–8.

8. Schlesinger PK, Donahue PE, Schmid B, et al. Limitations of 24-hour intraesophageal pH monitoring in the hospital setting. Gastroenterology 1985;89:797–804.

9. Zentilin P, Savarino V, Mastracci L, et al. Reassessment of the diagnostic value of histology in patients with GERD, using multiple biopsy sites and an appropriate control group. Am J Gastroenterol 2005;100:2299–306.

10. Gerson LB, Shetler K, Triadafilopoulos G. Prevalence of Barrett's esophagus in asymptomatic individuals. Gastroenterology 2002;123:461–7.

11. Finlay IG, Wright PA, Menzies T, et al. Microbial flora in carcinoma of oesophagus. Thorax 1982;37:181–4.

12. Bricard H, Deshayes JP, Sillard B, et al. Antibiotic prophylaxis in surgery of the esophagus. Ann Fr Anesth Reanim 1994;13:S161–8 [in French].

13. Gagliardi D, Makihara S, Corsi PR, et al. Microbial flora of the normal esophagus. Dis Esophagus 1998;11:248–50.

14. Mannell A, Plant M, Frolich J. The microflora of the oesophagus. Ann R Coll Surg Engl 1983;65:152–4.

15. Oliver JD. The viable but nonculturable state in bacteria. J Microbiol 2005; 43(Spec No):93–100.

16. Oliver JD. Recent findings on the viable but nonculturable state in pathogenic bacteria. FEMS Microbiol Rev 2010;34:415–25.

17. Weisburg WG, Barns SM, Pelletier DA, et al. 16S ribosomal DNA amplification for phylogenetic study. J Bacteriol 1991;173:697–703.

18. Pei Z, Bini EJ, Yang L, et al. Bacterial biota in the human distal esophagus. Proc Natl Acad Sci U S A 2004;101:4250–5.

19. Pei Z, Yang L, Peek RM Jr, et al. Bacterial biota in reflux esophagitis and Barrett's esophagus. World J Gastroenterol 2005;11:7277–83.

20. Yang L, Lu X, Nossa CW, et al. Inflammation and intestinal metaplasia of the distal esophagus are associated with alterations in the microbiome. Gastroenterology 2009;137:588–97.

21. Liu N, Ando T, Ishiguro K, et al. Characterization of bacterial biota in the distal esophagus of Japanese patients with reflux esophagitis and Barrett's esophagus. BMC Infect Dis 2013;13:130.

22. Gribar SC, Richardson WM, Sodhi CP, et al. No longer an innocent bystander: epithelial toll-like receptor signaling in the development of mucosal inflammation. Mol Med 2008;14:645–59.

23. Ioannou S, Voulgarelis M. Toll-like receptors, tissue injury, and tumourigenesis. Mediators Inflamm 2010;2010. pii:581837.

24. Mulder DJ, Lobo D, Mak N, et al. Expression of toll-like receptors 2 and 3 on esophageal epithelial cell lines and on eosinophils during esophagitis. Dig Dis Sci 2012;57:630–42.

25. Verbeek RE, Siersema PD, Ten Kate FJ, et al. Toll-like receptor 4 activation in Barrett's esophagus results in a strong increase in COX-2 expression. J Gastroenterol 2014;49(7):1121–34.

26. Wilson KT, Fu S, Ramanujam KS, et al. Increased expression of inducible nitric oxide synthase and cyclooxygenase-2 in Barrett's esophagus and associated adenocarcinomas. Cancer Res 1998;58:2929–34.

27. Shirvani VN, Ouatu-Lascar R, Kaur BS, et al. Cyclooxygenase 2 expression in Barrett's esophagus and adenocarcinoma: ex vivo induction by bile salts and acid exposure. Gastroenterology 2000;118:487–96.

28. Lim DM, Narasimhan S, Michaylira CZ, et al. TLR3-mediated NF-{kappa}B signaling in human esophageal epithelial cells. Am J Physiol Gastrointest Liver Physiol 2009;297:G1172–80.

29. Fitzgerald RC, Onwuegbusi BA, Bajaj-Elliott M, et al. Diversity in the oesophageal phenotypic response to gastro-oesophageal reflux: immunological determinants. Gut 2002;50:451–9.

30. Isomoto H, Saenko VA, Kanazawa Y, et al. Enhanced expression of interleukin-8 and activation of nuclear factor kappa-B in endoscopy-negative gastroesophageal reflux disease. Am J Gastroenterol 2004;99:589–97.

31. Isomoto H, Wang A, Mizuta Y, et al. Elevated levels of chemokines in esophageal mucosa of patients with reflux esophagitis. Am J Gastroenterol 2003;98:551–6.

32. Yoshida N, Uchiyama K, Kuroda M, et al. Interleukin-8 expression in the esophageal mucosa of patients with gastroesophageal reflux disease. Scand J Gastroenterol 2004;39:816–22.

33. Buttar NS, Wang KK, Leontovich O, et al. Chemoprevention of esophageal adenocarcinoma by COX-2 inhibitors in an animal model of Barrett's esophagus. Gastroenterology 2002;122:1101–12.

34. Oh DS, DeMeester SR, Vallbohmer D, et al. Reduction of interleukin 8 gene expression in reflux esophagitis and Barrett's esophagus with antireflux surgery. Arch Surg 2007;142:554–9 [discussion: 559–60].

35. O'Riordan JM, Abdel-latif MM, Ravi N, et al. Proinflammatory cytokine and nuclear factor kappa-B expression along the inflammation-metaplasia-dysplasia-adenocarcinoma sequence in the esophagus. Am J Gastroenterol 2005;100: 1257–64.

36. Isomoto H, Inoue K, Kohno S. Interleukin-8 levels in esophageal mucosa and long-term clinical outcome of patients with reflux esophagitis. Scand J Gastroenterol 2007;42:410–1.

37. Maeda S, Omata M. Inflammation and cancer: role of nuclear factor-kappaB activation. Cancer Sci 2008;99:836–42.

38. Souza RF, Krishnan K, Spechler SJ. Acid, bile, and CDX: the ABCs of making Barrett's metaplasia. Am J Physiol Gastrointest Liver Physiol 2008;295:G211–8.

39. Zhou X, Li D, Resnick MB, et al. NADPH oxidase NOX5-S and nuclear factor kappaB1 mediate acid-induced microsomal prostaglandin E synthase-1 expression in Barrett's esophageal adenocarcinoma cells. Mol Pharmacol 2013;83:978–90.

40. Huang B, Zhao J, Li H, et al. Toll-like receptors on tumor cells facilitate evasion of immune surveillance. Cancer Res 2005;65:5009–14.

41. Fan YP, Chakder S, Gao F, et al. Inducible and neuronal nitric oxide synthase involvement in lipopolysaccharide-induced sphincteric dysfunction. Am J Physiol Gastrointest Liver Physiol 2001;280:G32–42.

42. Hoshino K, Takeuchi O, Kawai T, et al. Cutting edge: toll-like receptor 4 (TLR4)-deficient mice are hyporesponsive to lipopolysaccharide: evidence for TLR4 as the Lps gene product. J Immunol 1999;162:3749–52.

43. Helminen O, Huhta H, Takala H, et al. Increased Toll-like receptor 5 expression indicates esophageal columnar dysplasia. Virchows Arch 2014;464:11–8.

44. Kauppila JH, Takala H, Selander KS, et al. Increased Toll-like receptor 9 expression indicates adverse prognosis in oesophageal adenocarcinoma. Histopathology 2011;59:643–9.

45. Hayashi F, Smith KD, Ozinsky A, et al. The innate immune response to bacterial flagellin is mediated by Toll-like receptor 5. Nature 2001;410:1099–103.
46. Hemmi H, Takeuchi O, Kawai T, et al. A Toll-like receptor recognizes bacterial DNA. Nature 2000;408:740–5.
47. Ding GC, Ren JL, Chang FB, et al. Human papillomavirus DNA and P16(INK4A) expression in concurrent esophageal and gastric cardia cancers. World J Gastroenterol 2010;16:5901–6.
48. Bosch FX, Lorincz A, Munoz N, et al. The causal relation between human papillomavirus and cervical cancer. J Clin Pathol 2002;55:244–65.
49. D'Souza G, Kreimer AR, Viscidi R, et al. Case-control study of human papillomavirus and oropharyngeal cancer. N Engl J Med 2007;356:1944–56.
50. Rajendra S, Robertson IK. Similar immunogenetics of Barrett's oesophagus and cervical neoplasia: is HPV the common denominator? J Clin Pathol 2010;63:1–3.
51. Rajendra S, Ackroyd R, Karim N, et al. Loss of human leucocyte antigen class I and gain of class II expression are early events in carcinogenesis: clues from a study of Barrett's oesophagus. J Clin Pathol 2006;59:952–7.
52. Wang X, Tian X, Liu F, et al. Detection of HPV DNA in esophageal cancer specimens from different regions and ethnic groups: a descriptive study. BMC Cancer 2010;10:19.
53. Rajendra S, Wang B, Snow ET, et al. Transcriptionally active human papillomavirus is strongly associated with Barrett's dysplasia and esophageal adenocarcinoma. Am J Gastroenterol 2013;108:1082–93.
54. Sedlak-Weinstein L, Remmerbach TW. Prevalence of HPV in suspicious oral lesions. The 47th Annual Scientific Meeting of the Australia and New Zealand Division of the International Association of Dental Research. Adelaide, Australia, September 8-12, 2007.
55. Gillison ML, Broutian T, Pickard RK, et al. Prevalence of oral HPV infection in the United States, 2009-2010. JAMA 2012;307:693–703.
56. Acevedo-Nuno E, Gonzalez-Ojeda A, Vazquez-Camacho G, et al. Human papillomavirus DNA and protein in tissue samples of oesophageal cancer, Barrett's oesophagus and oesophagitis. Anticancer Res 2004;24:1319–23.
57. Iyer A, Rajendran V, Adamson CS, et al. Human papillomavirus is detectable in Barrett's esophagus and esophageal carcinoma but is unlikely to be of any etiologic significance. J Clin Virol 2011;50:205–8.
58. El-Serag HB, Hollier JM, Gravitt P, et al. Human papillomavirus and the risk of Barrett's esophagus. Dis Esophagus 2013;26:517–21.
59. Kamath AM, Wu TT, Heitmiller R, et al. Investigation of the association of esophageal carcinoma with human papillomaviruses. Dis Esophagus 2000;13:122–4.
60. Rai N, Jenkins GJ, McAdam E, et al. Human papillomavirus infection in Barrett's oesophagus in the UK: an infrequent event. J Clin Virol 2008;43:250–2.
61. Tornesello ML, Monaco R, Nappi O, et al. Detection of mucosal and cutaneous human papillomaviruses in oesophagitis, squamous cell carcinoma and adenocarcinoma of the oesophagus. J Clin Virol 2009;45:28–33.
62. Morgan RJ, Perry AC, Newcomb PV, et al. Investigation of oesophageal adenocarcinoma for viral genomic sequences. Eur J Surg Oncol 1997;23:24–9.
63. Rokkas T, Pistiolas D, Sechopoulos P, et al. Relationship between *Helicobacter pylori* infection and esophageal neoplasia: a meta-analysis. Clin Gastroenterol Hepatol 2007;5:1413–7.
64. Islami F, Kamangar F. *Helicobacter pylori* and esophageal cancer risk: a meta-analysis. Cancer Prev Res (Phila) 2008;1:329–38.

65. Loffeld RJ, Werdmuller BF, Kuster JG, et al. Colonization with cagA-positive *Helicobacter pylori* strains inversely associated with reflux esophagitis and Barrett's esophagus. Digestion 2000;62:95–9.

66. Hamada H, Haruma K, Mihara M, et al. High incidence of reflux oesophagitis after eradication therapy for *Helicobacter pylori*: impacts of hiatal hernia and corpus gastritis. Aliment Pharmacol Ther 2000;14:729–35.

67. Peek RM. *Helicobacter pylori* and gastroesophageal reflux disease. Curr Treat Options Gastroenterol 2004;7:59–70.

68. Kado S, Uchida K, Funabashi H, et al. Intestinal microflora are necessary for development of spontaneous adenocarcinoma of the large intestine in T-cell receptor beta chain and p53 double-knockout mice. Cancer Res 2001;61: 2395–8.

69. Ley RE, Backhed F, Turnbaugh P, et al. Obesity alters gut microbial ecology. Proc Natl Acad Sci U S A 2005;102:11070–5.

70. Ferrer M, Martins dos Santos VA, Ott SJ, et al. Gut microbiota disturbance during antibiotic therapy: a multi-omic approach. Gut Microbes 2014;5:64–70.

71. Hayes RB, Reding D, Kopp W, et al. Etiologic and early marker studies in the prostate, lung, colorectal and ovarian (PLCO) cancer screening trial. Control Clin Trials 2000;21:349S–55S.

Microbiome in Human Immunodeficiency Virus Infection

January T. Salas, PhD, Theresa L. Chang, PhD*

KEYWORDS

- Microbiome • HIV transmission • HIV pathogenesis • Immune activation
- Microbial translocation

KEY POINTS

- Individuals infected with the human immunodeficiency virus (HIV) have altered microbiome associated with immune activation that impacts the consequence of disease progression.
- Genital and rectal microbiome may modulate the immune response and affect HIV transmission.

INTRODUCTION

Recent studies have demonstrated the important role of microbiota/microbiome in human health and diseases at cellular and molecular levels.[1–6] Interactions among microbes, nutrition, and immune response affect our health. For example, commensal bacteria protect the body from colonizing pathogenic bacteria by competing for space and nutrients.[7] Bacterial metabolites (ie, indole-3-aldehyde, butyric acid, hydrogen peroxide) could indirectly shape the host immune repertoire.[8,9] The advancement of techniques in sequencing and bioinformatics has made possible the characterization of microbial communities in health and diseased states. With this came an explosion of information shedding light on the important role of microbiota in the human body, from nutrition and autoimmunity to its role in brain diseases.[10]

An estimated 35.3 million people are living with human immunodeficiency virus (HIV) worldwide in addition to more than 2 million new cases since 2012 (UNAIDS 2013). Increasing evidence indicate that microbiome plays a crucial role in HIV transmission

This work was supported by National Institutes of Health R01AI110372.
The authors have nothing to disclose.
Department of Microbiology and Molecular Genetics, Public Health Research Institute, Rutgers-New Jersey Medical School, 225 Warren Street, Newark, NJ 07103, USA
* Corresponding author.
E-mail address: changth@njms.rutgers.edu

Clin Lab Med 34 (2014) 733–745
http://dx.doi.org/10.1016/j.cll.2014.08.005
0272-2712/14/$ – see front matter © 2014 Elsevier Inc. All rights reserved.
labmed.theclinics.com

and pathogenesis.[11–13] Alteration of vaginal and rectal microbiome may influence HIV acquisition[11,14–16] and mother-to-child transmission (MTCT).[17] The microbiome and immune response coevolve in response to infection during HIV pathogenesis that may determine the disease progression. Understanding the interplay between microbiome and HIV is vital for developing effective strategies for HIV prevention and treatment. This review summarizes the recent progress on microbiome in HIV transmission and pathogenesis. Although microbes are composed of bacteria, fungi, protozoa, and virus, the authors primarily focus on bacteria because of the availability of published data.

CHRONIC IMMUNE ACTIVATION IN HUMAN IMMUNODEFICIENCY VIRUS PATHOGENESIS

Persistent immune activation is a key feature of HIV, and markers of inflammation are a better predictor of clinical outcome than viral load.[18,19] Heightened immune activation and inflammation are associated with increased age-related diseases, such as cardiovascular, kidney, diabetes mellitus, and bone fracture, in patients with HIV.[20,21] Immune activation and inflammatory markers decline with antiretroviral therapy (ART) but always remain high compared with healthy controls.[22,23] Natural hosts of simian immunodeficiency virus (SIV), despite high viral loads, are able to avoid chronic infection through rapid controlled immune response and, hence, do not develop acquired immune deficiency syndrome (AIDS).[24–26]

Depletion of CD4+ T cells occurs within weeks after HIV infection, notably in the gut compartment.[27–30] Gut-associated interleukin-17 (IL-17) secreting CD4+ cells (Th17), important for mucosal defense against invading pathogens, are preferentially depleted.[31–33] Microbial translocation, translocation of microbes or microbial products without overt bacteremia, occurs after disruption of gut mucosal membrane integrity and mucosal immune homeostasis, which then could cause systemic immune activation.[18] Plasma lipopolysaccharide was elevated in HIV-infected patients and associated with an increase in plasma interferon α (IFNα) and frequency of activated CD8+ T cells (CD38+HLA-DR+).[18] Despite their activation status, only small portions of these CD8+ T cells are specific against HIV.[30] Additionally, expression of program death-1 on HIV-specific CD8+ T cells (marker also elevated in cytomegalovirus and Epstein-Barr virus infections) increases cell apoptosis and decreases their proliferative capacity.[34] Thus, in response to HIV infection, microbial translocation may cause chronic activation, leading to inflammatory-associated disease process and immune exhaustion. Note that the cause-and-effect relationship between microbial translocation and immune activation during chronic infection remains debatable despite several studies using animal models supporting the contribution of microbial translocation to immune activation (review in[21]). Although a recent study demonstrates early blockade of microbial translocation reduces inflammation and viral replication in SIV models,[35] the reciprocal interaction between microbial translocation and immune activation may contribute to SIV/HIV pathogenesis.

MICROBIOME SHAPES IMMUNE RESPONSE

Microbiota has major effects on immune cells and epithelial cells at the mucosa.[36] Mice raised in a clean facility, a condition that prevents natural colonization by microbiota, have increased mortality, bacteria burden on challenge, and susceptibility to infection compared with their counterparts raised in a conventional environment,[7,37] indicating the beneficial effects of early bacterial exposure on shaping host immunity.

For instance, *Lactobacillus casei* induces immunoglobulin A (IgA) and IL-6 producing cells in mouse gut lamina propia,[38] whereas segmented filamentous bacterium promotes the differentiation of Th17 cells in the gut.[39] In addition to the direct impact on immune response, microbes facilitate the processing and absorption of nutrients essential for immune functions, such as short fatty acids (butyrate and acetate) and amino acids (tryptophan).[40] Because different bacterial species induce different immune responses, the type of bacterial composition in the compartment could influence the balance between inflammation and homeostasis.[7]

Bacterial communities are diverse, and their compositions fluctuate with hormones, diet, and immune responses. They can be classified into 3 classes: (1) symbionts, bacteria known to promote health; (2) commensals, permanent residents with no known beneficial or detrimental effect to the host; and (3) pathobionts, permanent residents with the possibility to become pathogenic.[7] Patients with HIV infection or other diseases have alterations of microbial compositions.[41] Opportunistic pathogens, such as *Pseudomonas aeruginosa* and *Candida albicans*, are frequently found in HIV-infected patients who often have low to barely detectable levels of *Bifidobacteria* and *Lactobacilli* species in the gut.[42] *Bifidobacteria* and *Lactobacilli* are known to help improve gut health and immune function.[43,44] Prebiotics/probiotics supplements in patients with HIV on ART enhanced reconstitution of CD4+ T cells in the gastrointestinal tract, improved Th17 functionality, increased functionality and frequency of antigen presenting cells (APC), and decreased markers of immune activation. Likewise, an increase in *Prevotella* with decreased *Bacteroides* was associated with increased immune activation and microbial translocation.[12] Colonization of commensal *Lactobacillus crispatus*, *L jensenii*, and *L rhamnosus* on vaginal epithelial cell in vitro dampened inflammatory cytokine induction via toll-like receptor (TLR) activation.[36,45] Taken together, symbiotic/commensal bacteria modulate mucosal immune cells and maintain immune homeostasis. When symbiotic/commensal bacteria are compromised by overgrowth of indigenous pathobionts, leading to dysbiosis, immune cells will be activated to control pathogens. Immune activation and inflammation will result in collateral damage to the surrounding tissues.[7,37]

Bacterial metabolic products can modulate immune responses. For instance, the lack of butyric acid, a fermentation product from butyrate-producing bacteria in the gut, may lead to a decrease in regulatory T cells (Tregs) in inflammatory bowel disease.[46] In patients with HIV, enrichment of gut bacteria that catabolizes tryptophan, such as *Pseudomonas fluorescens*, inhibits Th17 cell differentiation and correlates with mucosal disruption.[47] Likewise, intestinal *Lactobacilli*, such as *L reuteri*, metabolize tryptophan to produce indole-3-aldehyde, which promotes IL-22 transcription.[8] Attachment of commensal *L crispatus* and *L jensenii* to the vaginal epithelium downregulates inflammatory cytokines, such as IL-6, tumor necrosis factor-α (TNF-α), and IL-8 on TLR-3 agonist polyinosinic/polycytidylic acid exposure, suggesting the immune-modulatory effect of colonization of commensal bacteria on epithelial cells.[36] This result indicates that the presence of commensal bacteria regulates the immune response of epithelial cells.

Changes in microbial communities in response to HIV/SIV infection and their association with immune activation have been recently documented.[14,18,26,42,47,48] HIV-infected patients given prebiotic/probiotic supplements exhibited reduced inflammation, enhanced CD4 reconstitution, and a subsequent improvement of prognosis, all highlighting the role of microbiota in HIV pathogenesis.[5] In the following sections, the authors summarize microbiome in various compartments in the context of HIV infection.

ORAL AND PERIODONTAL MICROBIOME

Oral lesions, frequently observed in HIV-positive patients without ART, are considered indicators of disease progression.[49] Oral lesions are often the first manifestation of HIV in places where the access to regular health care or ART is limited. Periodontal pathogens are more prevalent in HIV-infected individuals.[50] Oral microbial diversity with increased levels of total *Lactobacillus* species and *Candida* species was found to be greater in HIV-infected patients than uninfected controls.[41] Conversely, HIV-seropositive children have lower saliva bacterial species than uninfected children.[51] Macaques with infection by SIVmac251 intravenously had fewer oral bacterial species than uninfected animals followed by an outgrowth of *Gemella morbillorum*.[52] Certain microbial species are frequently found in HIV-infected patients but not in healthy individuals.[53] Preferential overgrowth of bacterial taxa, such *Candida spp*, *Gemella*, *Streptococcus*, *Veillonella*, and *Porphyromonas gingivalis*, in HIV-infected patients has been described.[28,48,49] Bacterial culture supernatant of *P gingivalis* reactivates HIV infection in cell lines with latent HIV proviruses through butyric acid-mediated histone acetylation and chromatin remodeling.[54] Elevated inflammatory cytokines, such as IL-6, IL-8, and granulocyte macrophage colony-stimulating factor, in periodontal pockets is observed in HIV-infected patients, which could be an immune response to opportunistic bacteria.[49]

ART decreases oral lesions, such as candidiasis in HIV-infected patients,[49,55] although the mechanism is not well defined. Reduction in viral load may have a direct impact on microbiota composition and oral epithelial cells. In monkeys, SIV downregulates the genes involved in oral epithelial regeneration, leading to slow healing of lesions.[56] A positive correlation between viral copies and bacterial growth has also been described.[48] In healthy rhesus macaques, *Streptococcus*, *Gemella*, and *Granulicatella* are 3 major genera in the lingual epithelium of the tongue dorsum, whereas *Streptococcus* and *Lachnospiraceae* are the core bacterial taxa in the dental plaque.[52] In response to intravenous SIV infection, there is a reduction of bacterial community diversity. Additionally, *Gemella* species became predominant; *Streptococcus* species were significantly reduced in the tongue dorsum. This dysbiosis is accompanied by the induction of IFNγ signaling pathways in tongue tissues. In vitro stimulation of oral epithelial cells with IFNγ results in the reduction of antimicrobial peptides, suggesting that SIV infection changes the microbial community through IFNγ-mediated downregulation of antimicrobial peptides.[52] The findings in SIV-infected macaques are similar to those in humans. *Streptococcus* is one of the predominant commensal genera in the human lingual epithelium.[57] The outgrown of *Gemella* species is also found in HIV-infected patients.[48] Specifically, *Gemella morbillorum* is a common opportunistic pathogen in HIV-infected patients with periodontitis.[28]

GUT MICROBIOME

Enteropathy is a common disorder in HIV-infected patients with AIDS.[58] Increasing evidence strongly indicates that HIV/SIV infection alters gut microbiome. Microbial analysis of colon biopsies reveals HIV-infected patients have more *Proteobacteria* and less *Firmicutes* than uninfected individuals.[12] Further analysis at a genus level showed an increase in *Prevotella* and a decrease in *Bacteroides* in HIV-infected patients. Alteration of the microbial community is accompanied by an increase in activation of colonic T cells and myeloid dendritic cells.[12] In chimpanzees, SIV infection alters gut microbial communities, which become more diverse over time.[59] The abundances of *Staphylococcus*, *Sarcina*, and *Selenomonas* were increased in response to infection.[59] Similarly, HIV-infected patients on ART with low viral loads have reduced populations of commensal bacteria that are replaced by bacterial communities, including *Brachyspira, Campylobacter, Catenibacterium, Escherichia, Enterobacteriaceae, Fusobacteriaceae, Mogibacterium, Prevotella*, and *Ralstonia*.[60] Total bacterial loads are similar among HIV-positive patients, HIV-positive patients on ART, and uninfected individuals. However, there is a difference in microbial compositions between HIV-positive patients and the uninfected group.[47] The HIV-positive group exhibited a profile of enriched pathobionts (ie, *Prevotella, Salmonella, Escherichia, Staphylococcus*, and *Campylobacter* species) accompanied reduced symbionts (ie, *Clostridia* and *Bacteroides*), a microbial profile referred to as disease-associated microbial communities (DMC).[47,60] Patients who are HIV positive on ART have an intermediate DMC profile between untreated HIV-positive patients and uninfected individuals. ART results in a shift in the DMC that resembles microbial communities in uninfected individuals. Studies of HIV-infected patients on ART, comparing partial immunologic responders (>200/μL CD4 count) and immunologic nonresponders (<200/μL), indicate that immunologic nonresponders have increased microbial translocation with elevated circulating 16S rDNA levels of more pathogenic *Enterobacteriaceae* and less of immunomodulatory *Lactobacillus* species.[61] Enrichment of genus *Prevotella* in HIV-positive patients was associated with increased immune activation and microbial translocation.[12] *Prevotella melaninogenica* enhanced HIV-1 expression in THP-1/NL4-3luc cells by the induction of TLR-2 in vitro.[62] Gut mucosal dysbiosis characterized by pathobionts, a common feature in HIV-infected individuals, is strongly associated with microbial translocation, immune activation, and viral persistence. The role of microbiome on the immune response in HIV-infected patients was demonstrated by the administration of probiotics/prebiotics in conjunction with ART leading to improved reconstitution of CD4 T cells, enhanced IL-23 secretion and number of APC, and increased the percentage of multifunctional Th17 cells in the gut.[5,44,63]

Altered microbiome in HIV-positive patients is also associated with high T-cell activation, plasma inflammation markers (IL-6, TNF), diminished mucosal IL-17– and IL-22–secreting cells, and increased tryptophan catabolism.[47,60] Diminished gut Th17 CD4+ T cells in HIV are thought to be the catalyst in the disruption of the mucosal barrier.[42] Indeed, Th17 cells are essential to mucosal homeostasis by orchestrating immune responses against invading pathogens and promoting mucosal barrier integrity through supporting the production of tight junction proteins and claudins.[64] Th17 cells are preferentially infected by HIV, leading to diminished numbers.[31–33] Recent evidence suggests gut microbiota may determine the fate of Th17 cells.[7,31] *Firmicutes*, a segmented filamentous bacterium, is essential for the development of Th17 cells.[39] By contrast, the gut bacteria *Pseudomonas fluorescens* is enriched in HIV-infected patients and has the capacity to catabolize tryptophan, generating catabolites that inhibit Th17 differentiation.[47] Indolamine-2,3-dioxygenase generated by myeloid dendritic cells catabolizes tryptophan to skew the differentiation of Tregs over Th17 cells.[9]

Gut microbiota provides the host the necessary nutrients and is critical in the development of a proper immune response.[65] A recent study by Shulzhenko and colleagues[2] reveals a bidirectional interaction between gut microbiota, mucosal epithelium, and gut-associated B cells whereby microbiota influences the balance between epithelial immune function and metabolic function. In the absence of IgA-secreting B cells, gut microbiota upregulates epithelial immune functions (upregulation IFN-induced genes and the complement system) at the expense of metabolic functions (downregulation of lipid, carbohydrate, and micronutrients related genes). Similarly, probiotic *Lactobacillus casei* administration to mice increased IgA-producing cells that were not specific to *L casei*.[38] Gene expression analysis of duodenal biopsies from HIV-infected patients reveals there is an upregulation of epithelial immune functions and a downregulation of epithelial metabolism, which could explain the malnutrition and malabsorption found in HIV-infected patients.[2] Taken together, microbiota/microbiome not only regulates the immune response but also nutrition and health in gut epithelium. It also modulates epithelial turnover, shedding, tight junctions, apoptosis, and autophagy.[66]

RECTAL MICROBIOME IN HUMAN IMMUNODEFICIENCY VIRUS

Rectal transmission is the main route of HIV transmission in men who have sex with men (MSM). In 2010, 78% of new infections were among MSM (Centers for Disease Control and Prevention). HIV infection is associated with a significant reduction in the diversity of microbial species in rectal mucosa; however, combined ART reverses this reduction to levels similar to healthy controls.[14] HIV-infected individuals have enrichment of *Fusobacteria, Anaerococcus, Peptostreptococcus*, and *Porphyromonas* with a depletion of *Roseburia, Ruminococcus, Eubacterium, Coprococcus*, and *Lachnospira*.[14] Analysis of metagenomic pathways demonstrated a downregulation of genes related to amino acid, fructose/mannose metabolism, and coenzyme A biosynthesis.[14] Similarly, as infection progressed in HIV-positive MSM, there was reduced alpha diversity and enrichment of *Fusobacteria*.[67]

Fusobacteria, enriched in HIV-infected individuals,[14,67] are abundant in the colorectal adenoma and associated with an increase in the local cytokine milieu suggestive of mucosal inflammation.[68] *Fusobacterium* isolated from ulcerative colitis secrete n-butyric acid,[69] a known histone deacetylase inhibitor (HDAC) that can reactivate latent HIV.[70,71] It remains to be determined whether enrichment of butyric acid producing *Fusobacteria* in rectal mucosa could increase HIV transmission.

VAGINAL AND CERVICAL MICROBIOME

Most studies that associate HIV with alterations of vaginal microbiota are performed in women diagnosed with bacterial vaginosis (BV),[72–74] which is a clinical symptom caused by an imbalance of commensal bacteria in the female genital tract. The predominant *Lactobacillus* species in the vagina are replaced by overgrowth of anaerobic bacteria, such as *Gardnerella, Atopobium, Prevotella*, and several other taxa.[72,73] A meta-analysis study comprising 23 publications with a total of 30,739 women clearly indicates an association between BV and an increased risk of HIV acquisition.[1] BV not only increases the risk of HIV acquisition but also transmission. HIV positive women with BV are greater than 3 times more likely to transmit HIV to their HIV-negative male partners than positive women without BV.[11] HIV MTCT was increased when there was alteration of vaginal microbiota to a *Gardnerella vaginalis* dominant species.[17] This finding clearly shows that the predominant community in a dysbiotic female reproductive tract alters the environment facilitating HIV entry and transmission.[75]

The vaginal microbiome comprises a dynamic ecosystem with important host defense capabilities that promote reproductive health. It is a kinetic ecosystem where the proportion of bacterial communities varies with hormonal changes, sexual activity, age, and race.[10,76] Nevertheless, the vaginal microbiome can be classified into 7 community types. Most of the vaginal communities, types I, II, III, and V, are dominated by one or more species of *Lactobacillus* that constitute most of all sequences obtained and are associated with a low vaginal pH (pH 4.0–5.0).[77] *Lactobacillus* dominance is lost in the type IV community, whereas *Gardnerella vaginalis* dominates the type VI community. Both types IV and VI are at higher risk for BV.[72,76] The type VII community has high, approximately even proportions of *G vaginalis* and *Lactobacillus* spp. *Lactobacilli* ferment glucose and produce lactic acid to maintain vaginal pH at an acidic state. The acidic pH environment is thought to prevent nonresident pathobionts from inhabiting and protects hosts against viral infection. H_2O_2-producing *Lactobacillus acidophilus* has an anti-HIV effect.[78] *Lactobacillus* species do not trigger proinflammatory cytokine production in vaginal epithelial cells, but nonresident skin bacteria *Staphylococcus epidermis* does.[36]

It is not clear how BV increases HIV acquisition and transmission; but it has been shown that BV increases viral shedding, increases the abundance of target cells, promotes the production of proinflammatory cytokines, and disrupts membrane integrity.[3,15,79–81] BV results in an increase in inflammatory cytokines[15] that remains present even during immunosuppressive states, such as pregnancy.[80] Also, high levels of inflammatory cytokines, such as IL-1β, IL-6, and IL-8, in cervicovaginal lavages (CVL) correlate with the reduction of CD4 T cells.[79] Furthermore, high concentrations of proinflammatory cytokines in CVL increased HIV-1 RNA levels and viral shedding.[81] *Atopobium vaginae*, not *L inners* or *L crispatus*, induce proinflammatory cytokines, antimicrobial peptides, and disrupt the mucosal barrier.[13] To summarize, vaginal dysbiosis in the setting of an inflammatory condition, such as BV, could increase HIV transmission by increasing target cells at the site, disrupting the mucosal barrier, and increasing viral shedding.

PENILE MICROBIOME IN HUMAN IMMUNODEFICIENCY VIRUS

Male circumcision reduces the incidences of urinary tract infection[6] and HIV acquisition.[82] Although the underlying mechanism remains to be defined, it is thought that penile foreskin, which is removed during circumcision, can trap HIV virions during sexual intercourse, increasing the opportunity for infection.[6] Additionally, the foreskin is lined with moist mucosal epithelium that provides an ideal environment for proinflammatory anaerobic bacteria and immune cells, such as Langerhans cells and CD4 T cells, target cells for HIV infection.[83] Foreskin inflammation manifested by massive infiltrates of CD4 and CD8 T cells increases HIV infection.[84] Male circumcision significantly reduces the bacterial load, the prevalence of some but not all anaerobic bacteria, and the microbiota diversity and composition.[85,86] Studies have clearly shown that circumcision reduces the risk of HIV acquisition and bacterial and viral sexually transmitted infections (STIs)[87,88]; however, the underlying mechanism remains to be defined.

LUNG MICROBIOME IN HUMAN IMMUNODEFICIENCY VIRUS

Bacterial pneumonia is frequently observed in HIV-positive patients.[89] Opportunistic infections in HIV-infected patients have been attributed to their state of immunosuppression. Bacterial rDNAs are detectable in lungs of HIV-infected individuals with no respiratory symptoms.[89] Bronchioalveolar lavage (BAL) of HIV-infected patients with pneumonia (from the San Francisco area) has a greater a number of taxa, including *Actinobacteria*, *Firmicutes*, *Cyanobacteria*, *Bacteroidetes*, and *Chloroflexi*, when compared with non-HIV patients with pneumonia.[90] On the other hand, HIV-infected patients (from a Uganda cohort) showed enrichment in members of *Lachnospiraceae* and sulfur-reducing bacteria (*Desulfovibrionaceae* and *Desulfuromonadaceae*) and exhibited even more diverse bacterial communities than the Western cohort.[91] The *Pseudomonas aeruginosa* pathogen was associated with pneumonia in the Uganda HIV cohort.[91] A metabolomics study of BAL from HIV-positive patients demonstrated increased levels of pyochelin metabolite, a by-product of *P aeruginosa*, which was not observed in healthy individuals.[92] HIV-infected patients have a high abundance of

Tropheryma whipplei, the causative agent of Whipple disease, in the lung, which is significantly reduced by ART.[4]

Diversity in lung microbiome between different cohorts of HIV-infected patients can be attributed to factors such as antimicrobial therapy, clinical status, ethnicity (genetics), diet, and environmental exposure.[91,93] Germ-free mice on challenge with ovalbumin exhibited exaggerated airway eosinophilia with increased production of IgE and Th2 cytokines compared with pathogen-free mice.[93] The contribution of environmental microbial exposures to HIV pathogenesis remains to be explored.

SUMMARY

HIV infection alters microbial communities in various mucosal compartments that may contribute to microbial translocation and immune activation during HIV disease progression. Conversely, microbiomes in the genital or rectal mucosa can impact the local immune response and HIV transmission. The bidirectional crosstalk between microbiome and the immune response may influence HIV transmission and pathogenesis. Further studies delineating the interplay between microbiome and immunity will offer insight into the development of a better strategy for HIV prevention and treatment.

REFERENCES

1. Atashili J, Poole C, Ndumbe PM, et al. Bacterial vaginosis and HIV acquisition: a meta-analysis of published studies. AIDS 2008;22(12):1493–501.
2. Shulzhenko N, Morgun A, Hsiao W, et al. Crosstalk between B lymphocytes, microbiota and the intestinal epithelium governs immunity versus metabolism in the gut. Nat Med 2011;17(12):1585–93.
3. Petrova MI, van den Broek M, Balzarini J, et al. Vaginal microbiota and its role in HIV transmission and infection. FEMS Microbiol Rev 2013;37(5):762–92.
4. Lozupone C, Cota-Gomez A, Palmer BE, et al. Widespread colonization of the lung by Tropheryma whipplei in HIV infection. Am J Respir Crit Care Med 2013;187(10):1110–7.
5. Klatt NR, Canary LA, Sun X, et al. Probiotic/prebiotic supplementation of antiretrovirals improves gastrointestinal immunity in SIV-infected macaques. J Clin Invest 2013;123(2):903–7.
6. Anderson D, Politch JA, Pudney J. HIV infection and immune defense of the penis. Am J Reprod Immunol 2011;65(3):220–9.
7. Round JL, Mazmanian SK. The gut microbiota shapes intestinal immune responses during health and disease. Nat Rev Immunol 2009;9(5):313–23.
8. Zelante T, Iannitti RG, Cunha C, et al. Tryptophan catabolites from microbiota engage aryl hydrocarbon receptor and balance mucosal reactivity via interleukin-22. Immunity 2013;39(2):372–85.
9. Favre D, Mold J, Hunt PW, et al. Tryptophan catabolism by indoleamine 2,3-dioxygenase 1 alters the balance of TH17 to regulatory T cells in HIV disease. Sci Transl Med 2010;2(32):32ra36.
10. Human Microbiome Project Consortium. Structure, function and diversity of the healthy human microbiome. Nature 2012;486(7402):207–14.
11. Cohen CR, Lingappa JR, Baeten JM, et al. Bacterial vaginosis associated with increased risk of female-to-male HIV-1 transmission: a prospective cohort analysis among African couples. PLoS Med 2012;9(6):e1001251.
12. Dillon SM, Lee EJ, Kotter CV, et al. An altered intestinal mucosal microbiome in HIV-1 infection is associated with mucosal and systemic immune activation and endotoxemia. Mucosal Immunol 2014;7(4):983–94.

13. Doerflinger SY, Throop AL, Herbst-Kralovetz MM. Bacteria in the vaginal microbiome alter the innate immune response and barrier properties of the human vaginal epithelia in a species-specific manner. J Infect Dis 2014;209(12): 1989–99.

14. McHardy IH, Li X, Tong M, et al. HIV Infection is associated with compositional and functional shifts in the rectal mucosal microbiota. Microbiome 2013; 1(1):26.

15. Sturm-Ramirez K, Gaye-Diallo A, Eisen G, et al. High levels of tumor necrosis factor-alpha and interleukin-1beta in bacterial vaginosis may increase susceptibility to human immunodeficiency virus. J Infect Dis 2000;182(2):467–73.

16. Martin HL, Richardson BA, Nyange PM, et al. Vaginal lactobacilli, microbial flora, and risk of human immunodeficiency virus type 1 and sexually transmitted disease acquisition. J Infect Dis 1999;180(6):1863–8.

17. Frank DN, Manigart O, Leroy V, et al. Altered vaginal microbiota are associated with perinatal mother-to-child transmission of HIV in African women from Burkina Faso. J Acquir Immune Defic Syndr 2012;60(3):299–306.

18. Brenchley JM, Price DA, Schacker TW, et al. Microbial translocation is a cause of systemic immune activation in chronic HIV infection. Nat Med 2006;12(12): 1365–71.

19. Hunt PW. HIV and inflammation: mechanisms and consequences. Curr HIV/ AIDS Rep 2012;9(2):139–47.

20. Guaraldi G, Orlando G, Zona S, et al. Premature age-related comorbidities among HIV-infected persons compared with the general population. Clin Infect Dis 2011;53(11):1120–6.

21. Marchetti G, Tincati C, Silvestri G. Microbial translocation in the pathogenesis of HIV infection and AIDS. Clin Microbiol Rev 2013;26(1):2–18.

22. Hazenberg MD, Stuart JW, Otto SA, et al. T-cell division in human immunodeficiency virus (HIV)-1 infection is mainly due to immune activation: a longitudinal analysis in patients before and during highly active antiretroviral therapy (HAART). Blood 2000;95(1):249–55.

23. Neuhaus J, Jacobs DR Jr, Baker JV, et al. Markers of inflammation, coagulation, and renal function are elevated in adults with HIV infection. J Infect Dis 2010; 201(12):1788–95.

24. Brenchley JM, Silvestri G, Douek DC. Nonprogressive and progressive primate immunodeficiency lentivirus infections. Immunity 2010;32(6):737–42.

25. Jacquelin B, Mayau V, Targat B, et al. Nonpathogenic SIV infection of African green monkeys induces a strong but rapidly controlled type I IFN response. J Clin Invest 2009;119(12):3544–55.

26. Silvestri G, Sodora DL, Koup RA, et al. Nonpathogenic SIV infection of sooty mangabeys is characterized by limited bystander immunopathology despite chronic high-level viremia. Immunity 2003;18(3):441–52.

27. Lim SG, Condez A, Lee CA, et al. Loss of mucosal CD4 lymphocytes is an early feature of HIV infection. Clin Exp Immunol 1993;92(3):448–54.

28. Aas JA, Barbuto SM, Alpagot T, et al. Subgingival plaque microbiota in HIV positive patients. J Clin Periodontol 2007;34(3):189–95.

29. Veazey RS, DeMaria M, Chalifoux LV, et al. Gastrointestinal tract as a major site of CD4+ T cell depletion and viral replication in SIV infection. Science 1998; 280(5362):427–31.

30. Brenchley JM, Schacker TW, Ruff LE, et al. CD4+ T cell depletion during all stages of HIV disease occurs predominantly in the gastrointestinal tract. J Exp Med 2004;200(6):749–59.

31. Blaschitz C, Raffatellu M. Th17 cytokines and the gut mucosal barrier. J Clin Immunol 2010;30(2):196–203.

32. Raffatellu M, Santos RL, Verhoeven DE, et al. Simian immunodeficiency virus-induced mucosal interleukin-17 deficiency promotes Salmonella dissemination from the gut. Nat Med 2008;14(4):421–8.

33. Brenchley JM, Paiardini M, Knox KS, et al. Differential Th17 CD4 T-cell depletion in pathogenic and nonpathogenic lentiviral infections. Blood 2008;112(7):2826–35.

34. Petrovas C, Casazza JP, Brenchley JM, et al. PD-1 is a regulator of virus-specific CD8+ T cell survival in HIV infection. J Exp Med 2006;203(10):2281–92.

35. Kristoff J, Haret-Richter G, Ma D, et al. Early microbial translocation blockade reduces SIV-mediated inflammation and viral replication. J Clin Invest 2014; 124(6):2802–6.

36. Rose WA 2nd, McGowin CL, Spagnuolo RA, et al. Commensal bacteria modulate innate immune responses of vaginal epithelial cell multilayer cultures. PLoS One 2012;7(3):e32728.

37. Cerf-Bensussan N, Gaboriau-Routhiau V. The immune system and the gut microbiota: friends or foes? Nat Rev Immunol 2010;10(10):735–44.

38. Galdeano CM, Perdigon G. The probiotic bacterium Lactobacillus casei induces activation of the gut mucosal immune system through innate immunity. Clin Vaccine Immunol 2006;13(2):219–26.

39. Ivanov II, Atarashi K, Manel N, et al. Induction of intestinal Th17 cells by segmented filamentous bacteria. Cell 2009;139(3):485–98.

40. Kau AL, Ahern PP, Griffin NW, et al. Human nutrition, the gut microbiome and the immune system. Nature 2011;474(7351):327–36.

41. Saxena D, Li Y, Yang L, et al. Human microbiome and HIV/AIDS. Curr HIV/AIDS Rep 2012;9(1):44–51.

42. Gori A, Tincati C, Rizzardini G, et al. Early impairment of gut function and gut flora supporting a role for alteration of gastrointestinal mucosa in human immunodeficiency virus pathogenesis. J Clin Microbiol 2008;46(2):757–8.

43. Saavedra JM, Bauman NA, Oung I, et al. Feeding of Bifidobacterium bifidum and Streptococcus thermophilus to infants in hospital for prevention of diarrhoea and shedding of rotavirus. Lancet 1994;344(8929):1046–9.

44. Hummelen R, Changalucha J, Butamanya NL, et al. Effect of 25 weeks probiotic supplementation on immune function of HIV patients. Gut Microbes 2011;2(2): 80–5.

45. Pyles RB, Vincent KL, Baum MM, et al. Cultivated vaginal microbiomes alter HIV-1 infection and antiretroviral efficacy in colonized epithelial multilayer cultures. PLoS One 2014;9(3):e93419.

46. Furusawa Y, Obata Y, Fukuda S, et al. Commensal microbe-derived butyrate induces the differentiation of colonic regulatory T cells. Nature 2013;504(7480): 446–50.

47. Vujkovic-Cvijin I, Dunham RM, Iwai S, et al. Dysbiosis of the gut microbiota is associated with HIV disease progression and tryptophan catabolism. Sci Transl Med 2013;5(193):193ra191.

48. Dang AT, Cotton S, Sankaran-Walters S, et al. Evidence of an increased pathogenic footprint in the lingual microbiome of untreated HIV infected patients. BMC Microbiol 2012;12:153.

49. Ryder MI. Periodontal management of HIV-infected patients. Periodontol 2000 2000;23:85–93.

50. Pereira VT, Pavan P, Souza RC, et al. The association between detectable plasmatic human immunodeficiency virus (HIV) viral load and different subgingival

microorganisms in Brazilian adults with HIV: a multilevel analysis. J Periodontol 2014;85(5):697–705.

51. Silva-Boghossian C, Castro GF, Teles RP, et al. Salivary microbiota of HIV-positive children and its correlation with HIV status, oral diseases, and total secretory IgA. Int J Paediatr Dent 2008;18(3):205–16.

52. Ocon S, Murphy C, Dang AT, et al. Transcription profiling reveals potential mechanisms of dysbiosis in the oral microbiome of rhesus macaques with chronic untreated SIV infection. PLoS One 2013;8(11):e80863.

53. Mataftsi M, Skoura L, Sakellari D. HIV infection and periodontal diseases: an overview of the post-HAART era. Oral Dis 2011;17(1):13–25.

54. Imai K, Ochiai K, Okamoto T. Reactivation of latent HIV-1 infection by the periodontopathic bacterium Porphyromonas gingivalis involves histone modification. J Immunol 2009;182(6):3688–95.

55. Greenspan D, Gange SJ, Phelan JA, et al. Incidence of oral lesions in HIV-1-infected women: reduction with HAART. J Dent Res 2004;83(2):145–50.

56. George MD, Verhoeven D, Sankaran S, et al. Heightened cytotoxic responses and impaired biogenesis contribute to early pathogenesis in the oral mucosa of simian immunodeficiency virus-infected rhesus macaques. Clin Vaccine Immunol 2009;16(2):277–81.

57. Aas JA, Paster BJ, Stokes LN, et al. Defining the normal bacterial flora of the oral cavity. J Clin Microbiol 2005;43(11):5721–32.

58. Kotler DP, Gaetz HP, Lange M, et al. Enteropathy associated with the acquired immunodeficiency syndrome. Ann Intern Med 1984;101(4):421–8.

59. Moeller AH, Shilts M, Li Y, et al. SIV-induced instability of the chimpanzee gut microbiome. Cell Host Microbe 2013;14(3):340–5.

60. Mutlu EA, Keshavarzian A, Losurdo J, et al. A compositional look at the human gastrointestinal microbiome and immune activation parameters in HIV infected subjects. PLoS Pathog 2014;10(2):e1003829.

61. Merlini E, Bai F, Bellistri GM, et al. Evidence for polymicrobic flora translocating in peripheral blood of HIV-infected patients with poor immune response to antiretroviral therapy. PLoS One 2011;6(4):e18580.

62. Ahmed N, Hayashi T, Hasegawa A, et al. Suppression of human immunodeficiency virus type 1 replication in macrophages by commensal bacteria preferentially stimulating Toll-like receptor 4. J Gen Virol 2010;91(Pt 11): 2804–13.

63. Perez-Santiago J, Gianella S, Massanella M, et al. Gut Lactobacillales are associated with higher CD4 and less microbial translocation during HIV infection. AIDS 2013;27(12):1921–31.

64. Dandekar S, George MD, Baumler AJ. Th17 cells, HIV and the gut mucosal barrier. Curr Opin HIV AIDS 2010;5(2):173–8.

65. Smith PM, Garrett WS. The gut microbiota and mucosal T cells. Front Microbiol 2011;2:111.

66. Kim M, Ashida H, Ogawa M, et al. Bacterial interactions with the host epithelium. Cell Host Microbe 2010;8(1):20–35.

67. Yu G, Fadrosh D, Ma B, et al. Anal microbiota profiles in HIV-positive and HIV-negative MSM. AIDS 2014;28(5):753–60.

68. McCoy AN, Araujo-Perez F, Azcarate-Peril A, et al. Fusobacterium is associated with colorectal adenomas. PLoS One 2013;8(1):e53653.

69. Ohkusa T, Okayasu I, Ogihara T, et al. Induction of experimental ulcerative colitis by Fusobacterium varium isolated from colonic mucosa of patients with ulcerative colitis. Gut 2003;52(1):79–83.

70. Shirakawa K, Chavez L, Hakre S, et al. Reactivation of latent HIV by histone deacetylase inhibitors. Trends Microbiol 2013;21(6):277–85.

71. Victoriano AF, Imai K, Okamoto T. Interaction between endogenous bacterial flora and latent HIV infection. Clin Vaccine Immunol 2013;20(6):773–9.

72. Hummelen R, Fernandes AD, Macklaim JM, et al. Deep sequencing of the vaginal microbiota of women with HIV. PLoS One 2010;5(8):e12078.

73. Spear GT, Gilbert D, Sikaroodi M, et al. Identification of rhesus macaque genital microbiota by 16S pyrosequencing shows similarities to human bacterial vaginosis: implications for use as an animal model for HIV vaginal infection. AIDS Res Hum Retroviruses 2010;26(2):193–200.

74. Spear GT, Sikaroodi M, Zariffard MR, et al. Comparison of the diversity of the vaginal microbiota in HIV-infected and HIV-uninfected women with or without bacterial vaginosis. J Infect Dis 2008;198(8):1131–40.

75. Schellenberg JJ, Plummer FA. The microbiological context of HIV resistance: vaginal microbiota and mucosal inflammation at the viral point of entry. Int J Inflam 2012;2012:131243.

76. Gajer P, Brotman RM, Bai G, et al. Temporal dynamics of the human vaginal microbiota. Sci Transl Med 2012;4(132):132ra152.

77. Ravel J, Gajer P, Abdo Z, et al. Vaginal microbiome of reproductive-age women. Proc Natl Acad Sci U S A 2011;108(Suppl 1):4680–7.

78. Klebanoff SJ, Coombs RW. Viricidal effect of Lactobacillus acidophilus on human immunodeficiency virus type 1: possible role in heterosexual transmission. J Exp Med 1991;174(1):289–92.

79. Bebell LM, Passmore JA, Williamson C, et al. Relationship between levels of inflammatory cytokines in the genital tract and CD4+ cell counts in women with acute HIV-1 infection. J Infect Dis 2008;198(5):710–4.

80. Beigi RH, Yudin MH, Cosentino L, et al. Cytokines, pregnancy, and bacterial vaginosis: comparison of levels of cervical cytokines in pregnant and nonpregnant women with bacterial vaginosis. J Infect Dis 2007;196(9):1355–60.

81. Mitchell C, Hitti J, Paul K, et al. Cervicovaginal shedding of HIV type 1 is related to genital tract inflammation independent of changes in vaginal microbiota. AIDS Res Hum Retroviruses 2011;27(1):35–9.

82. Auvert B, Taljaard D, Lagarde E, et al. Randomized, controlled intervention trial of male circumcision for reduction of HIV infection risk: the ANRS 1265 Trial. PLoS Med 2005;2(11):e298.

83. Price LB, Liu CM, Johnson KE, et al. The effects of circumcision on the penis microbiome. PLoS One 2010;5(1):e8422.

84. Johnson KE, Sherman ME, Ssempiija V, et al. Foreskin inflammation is associated with HIV and herpes simplex virus type-2 infections in Rakai, Uganda. AIDS 2009;23(14):1807–15.

85. Liu CM, Hungate BA, Tobian AA, et al. Male circumcision significantly reduces prevalence and load of genital anaerobic bacteria. MBio 2013;4(2):e00076.

86. Schneider JA, Vadivelu S, Liao C, et al. Increased likelihood of bacterial pathogens in the coronal sulcus and urethra of uncircumcised men in a diverse group of HIV infected and uninfected patients in India. J Glob Infect Dis 2012;4(1):6–9.

87. Corey L, Wald A, Celum CL, et al. The effects of herpes simplex virus-2 on HIV-1 acquisition and transmission: a review of two overlapping epidemics. J Acquir Immune Defic Syndr 2004;35(5):435–45.

88. Weiss HA, Thomas SL, Munabi SK, et al. Male circumcision and risk of syphilis, chancroid, and genital herpes: a systematic review and meta-analysis. Sex Transm Infect 2006;82(2):101–9 [discussion: 110].

89. Segal LN, Methe BA, Nolan A, et al. HIV-1 and bacterial pneumonia in the era of antiretroviral therapy. Proc Am Thorac Soc 2011;8(3):282–7.
90. Iwai S, Fei M, Huang D, et al. Oral and airway microbiota in HIV-infected pneumonia patients. J Clin Microbiol 2012;50(9):2995–3002.
91. Iwai S, Huang D, Fong S, et al. The lung microbiome of Ugandan HIV-infected pneumonia patients is compositionally and functionally distinct from that of San Franciscan patients. PLoS One 2014;9(4):e95726.
92. Cribbs SK, Park Y, Guidot DM, et al. Metabolomics of bronchoalveolar lavage differentiate healthy HIV-1-infected subjects from controls. AIDS Res Hum Retroviruses 2014;30(6):579–85.
93. Beck JM, Young VB, Huffnagle GB. The microbiome of the lung. Transl Res 2012;160(4):258–66.

The Changing Landscape of the Vaginal Microbiome

Bernice Huang, PhD[a], Jennifer M. Fettweis, PhD[a], J. Paul Brooks, PhD[b],
Kimberly K. Jefferson, PhD[a], Gregory A. Buck, PhD[a,*]

KEYWORDS

- Vaginal microbiome • Pregnancy • Bacterial vaginosis • Preterm birth
- Metagenomics • Microbiota

KEY POINTS

- The vaginal microenvironment is a dynamic ecosystem in which the microbiota play a major role in regulating parameters such as pH and in limiting the growth of potentially harmful organisms.
- Alterations in the vaginal microbiota can impact the community's ability to inhibit pathogenesis of disease-causing organisms in the female urogenital tract.
- Bacterial vaginosis is broadly, but apparently only poorly, defined by the disruption of the normal vaginal ecosystem marked by depletion of lactobacilli and overgrowth of anaerobic bacteria.

INTRODUCTION

The microbiome influences humans in many still underappreciated respects, including, but not limited to, development and growth, immunity, metabolism, and even behavior.[1,2] Most bacterial communities exist in mutualistic relationships with the healthy human host, and it is clear that our microbiota evolved in concert with our genome, the product of which is a true human–microbial symbiosis. However, it is also clear that microbial dysbiosis can result in disease, and the outgrowth of opportunistic pathogens can threaten the health and life of the human host. Fueled in part by the Human Microbiome Project (HMP) of the National Institutes of Health (NIH) and

The authors have nothing to disclose.
This work was supported by National Institutes of Health grants 4UH3AI083263, The Vaginal Microbiome: Disease, Genetics and the Environment, and 8U54HD080784 Multi-omic Analysis of the Vaginal Microbiome During Pregnancy (MOMS-PI).
[a] Department of Microbiology and Immunology, Center for the Study of Biological Complexity, 1101 East Marshall Street, PO Box 980678, Richmond, VA 23298, USA; [b] Department of Statistical Sciences and Operations Research, Virginia Commonwealth University, PO Box 843083, Richmond, VA 23284, USA
* Corresponding author.
E-mail address: gabuck@vcu.edu

similar efforts by other groups worldwide,[3–5] large-scale efforts have been made to define the normal microbiome of healthy individuals across multiple body sites. Facilitated by the advent of next-generation sequencing, a major success of the first phase of these efforts has been the wealth of data generated, which collectively has revealed the previously poorly recognized complexity and dynamic nature of the human microbiome and its stunning impacts on human health and well-being. To further explore the functional role of the microbiome in human health and disease, the NIH has launched HMP2, now termed the *integrative* HMP or iHMP, a second phase of study that mandates a more in-depth "multi-omic" approach to explore host–bacterial interactions and community dynamics in the context of human health and disease.

The Vaginal Microbiome Consortium (vmc.vcu.edu) at Virginia Commonwealth University (VCU) has a two-stage project funded by the NIH HMP1 and iHMP programs. The first stage, the Vaginal Human Microbiome Project, is a cross-sectional community-based study on more than 6000 visitors to multiple women's clinics in Central Virginia, with the goal of investigating the roles of the vaginal microbiome in women's urogenital health. Vaginal and buccal samples were collected from women volunteers older than 18 years, with the exception of women who were incarcerated, independent of their state of health. Embedded within this study is the collection and analysis of samples from approximately 250 monozygotic and dizygotic twin pairs from VCU's Mid-Atlantic Twin Registry.[6] The microbial populations in each sample were defined by high-throughput metagenomic 16S rRNA gene sequencing, whole metagenome shotgun analysis, and by microbiologically culturing, cloning by single colony isolation, and sequencing of the genomes of target bacterial species or taxa. In the Multi-Omic Microbiome Study-Pregnancy Initiative, the second stage of this program, samples from more than 2000 pregnant women and their infants are being collected longitudinally at multiple prenatal visits during their pregnancies, at delivery, and at early postnatal visits. Samples are collected from the vagina, rectum, nares, mouth and skin from each participant older than 15 years who is not incarcerated and who is not a surrogate.

Samples from these participants are subjected to six omics technologies: (1) targeted 16S rRNA gene surveys to generate species-level microbiome profiles; (2) whole genome sequencing of relevant taxa that we are able to culture and bacteriologically clone; (3) whole metagenomic shotgun sequencing to generate "gene-centric" and "taxonomy-centric" profiles of the metabolic and pathogenic potential, and to generate genome sequences of abundant taxa that we are unable to cultivate; (4) metatranscriptomic analysis to assess expression levels of relevant prokaryotic and host genes; (5) metabolomic/lipidomic analyses to provide insight into the signaling and regulatory pathways controlling the environment in the vagina; and (6) immunoproteomic analyses to measure cytokines and immune factors impacting vaginal function during pregnancy. The objective of the latter study is to elucidate the role(s) of the vaginal microbiome in the etiology or prevention of adverse outcomes of pregnancy, with a specific focus on preterm birth (PTB) and stillbirth.

THE VAGINAL MICROBIOME

Microbial communities play fundamental roles in promoting homeostasis in the vagina and in preventing colonization of pathogenic bacteria, but the mechanisms by which they exert their influence are not well defined. Historically, studies of vaginal microbiota applied conventional culture-dependent microbiological strategies, which, because most of the microbial species in these environments are intractable to standard cultivation technologies, produce only a partial picture of the overall microbiome.

Development of culture-independent approaches based on analysis of 16S rRNA gene sequences, coupled with the establishment of high-throughput so-called next-generation sequencing technology,[7] now permits deep, high-resolution, species-level classification[8] of vaginally relevant bacteria and is dramatically broadening our understanding of the vaginal ecosystem and the complex interactions between host and microbial factors within it.

Since their first description in 1892 by Gustav Doderlein, lactobacilli have been considered the dominant inhabitants of vaginal communities and the cornerstone of vaginal health.[9] The prevailing hypothesis holds that vaginal *Lactobacillus* species promote a protective environment in the vagina by lowering the pH through lactic acid production and by competing for nutrients and space. *Lactobacillus* species also produce other metabolites, bacteriocins and hydrogen peroxide (H_2O_2), which may contribute to the inhibition of growth of other microorganisms[10,11] and therefore have the potential to actively protect the vaginal ecosystem from adverse microbiota.

Recent studies have produced major advances in our understanding of the composition of vaginal microbial communities. Collectively, this research has revealed the presence of several distinct types of communities that differ in both the composition and relative abundance of species or taxa. The prevalence of these communities varies significantly among different racial and ethnic groups.[12–14] This observation is important because differences in microbial composition may radically influence how vaginal communities respond to infections or other imbalances. Here, we review studies of the vaginal microbiome, including factors that influence its composition and its role in the maintenance of vaginal health.

HEALTHY *LACTOBACILLUS*-DOMINATED VAGINAL FLORA

The genus *Lactobacillus* comprises more than 130 lactic acid–producing species that inhabit diverse environments; over 20 of which have been detected in the vagina.[15,16] Unlike most other body sites, healthy vaginal communities were considered to be those dominated by only one or two species, the most common of which are *Lactobacillus iners*, *Lactobacillus crispatus*, *Lactobacillus jensenii* and *Lactobacillus gasseri*.[12,17] Lactobacilli use several mechanisms to inhibit colonization by other bacteria, including pathogens. Vaginal epithelial cells produce glycogen, which lactobacilli ferment, producing D- and L-lactic acid.[18] Some species produce hydrogen peroxide in vitro; however, recent studies suggest that in the hypoxic conditions that exist in the vagina, concentrations may never achieve levels that are inhibitory to other bacteria.[19] In vaginal fluid, bacteria associated with bacterial vaginosis can be suppressed with lactic acid but not hydrogen peroxide.[20,21] Some species also produce bacteriocins that can directly kill other bacterial species.[22] Lactobacilli also likely out compete other organisms for nutrients or receptors at the epithelial cell surface.[23–25] These inhibitory mechanisms differ among *Lactobacillus* species. Comparative genomic analyses of *L crispatus*, *L gasseri*, *L iners* and *L jensenii* have provided evidence that each *Lactobacillus* species possesses a unique repertoire of protein families and suggest these differences may reflect specific community adaptations.[26,27] Future studies aimed at characterizing the functional roles of these species-specific protein families and genes may provide important insight into how these common vaginal bacteria impact women's health.

Lactobacilli can also inhibit pathogen colonization by competing for host cell receptors used by urogenital pathogens such as *Gardnerella vaginalis*, *Neisseria gonorrhoeae*, *Candida albicans*, *Staphylococcus aureus*, group B *Streptococcus* species, *Pseudomonas aeruginosa*, *Streptococcus agalactiae*, *Escherichia coli* and *Prevotella bivia*.[23,28–30] Thus, lactobacilli with a higher affinity for host cell receptors can displace adherent *G vaginalis* and *N gonorrhoeae*.[25,31] Furthermore, some lactobacilli are thought to co-aggregate with pathogens (eg, *G vaginalis*, *C albicans* and *E coli*), thereby inhibiting them from binding to host cells and allowing more effective clearance.[32,33]

From the host perspective, several factors, including, but not limited to, the periodic hormonal cycling that promotes release of glycogen into the vaginal environment and the continual sloughing of the epithelial cells to which bacteria are attached, contribute to innate defenses against pathogen colonization. Presumably, the collective activities of the host, in concert with inhibitory mechanisms of *Lactobacillus*, contribute to the maintenance of a healthy vaginal ecosystem.

HEALTHY NON-*LACTOBACILLUS*—DOMINATED VAGINAL FLORA

Although a prevalence of *Lactobacillus* species is the most common signature of a healthy microbiome, a significant proportion of apparently healthy women have vaginal bacterial communities that lack appreciable numbers of *Lactobacillus* species but include a diverse range of facultative or strictly anaerobic bacteria that are typically associated with slightly elevated pH. These microbiota include members of the genera *Atopobium*, *Corynebacterium*, *Anaerococcus*, *Peptoniphilus*, *Prevotella*, *Mobiluncus*, *Gardnerella* and *Sneathia*, bacteria that are usually associated with a dysbiotic or diseased state.[12,14,16,34–36] Some of these bacteria, such as *Atopobium* can also produce lactic acid.[37] Thus, the question remains whether certain bacterial taxa can play the role as either healthy commensal or pathogen, depending on other factors.

FACTORS THAT INFLUENCE THE MICROBIOME

Many factors influence the stability of the vaginal microbiota. The composition of vaginal communities fluctuates as a function of age, menarche, menses, pregnancy, infections, birth control and sexual behaviors.[17,38–41] Exposure to spermicides or β-lactam or other antimicrobials can decrease the prevalence of lactobacilli and consequently increase susceptibility to vaginal infections.[42,43]

Acquisition of the vaginal microbiome occurs shortly after or during birth. In utero, the fetus was once thought to exist in a sterile or near-sterile environment, but several culture-independent studies now suggest the placental microbiome harbors low-abundance microbial communities.[44–46] With a vaginal delivery, the neonate is exposed to a diverse array of microbes, including those encountered during passage through the mother's birth canal. Culture-based studies in humans suggest that neonates acquire their initial microbiota from the vagina and feces of their mothers.[47] Dominguez-Bello and colleagues[48] used targeted 16S rRNA gene sequencing to show that vaginally delivered infants (n = 4) acquire microbial communities across skin, oral, nasopharyngeal and gut habitats similar to the vaginal microbiota of their mother, most commonly dominated by *Lactobacillus*, *Prevotella*, or *Sneathia* spp., whereas cesarean section–delivered infants (n = 6) acquire microbial communities similar to those inhabiting their mother's skin, dominated by *Staphylococcus*, *Corynebacterium* and *Propionibacterium* spp. Other studies have found that meconium of full-term infants harbor bacteria,[49,50] indicating that gut colonization is seeded before birth. Additional studies have reported that the gastrointestinal tracts of vaginally delivered newborns acquire several strains of *Bifidobacterium* from the intestine of the mother, suggesting that delivery mode and the mother's intestinal microbiota are key factors in establishing the infant's intestinal microbiota during early infancy.[51,52] It remains unclear how differences in the mode of delivery will impact development of the infant microbiome over time and what, if any, the subsequent effects on health will be.

Changes in the composition of the vaginal flora are driven by the dramatic hormonal shifts that occur throughout a woman's life. During early childhood, the vaginal pH is neutral or only slightly alkaline.[53–55] As estrogen levels increase during puberty, increased amounts of glycogen deposited in the vaginal epithelium permits the ascendance and eventual predominance of lactic acid–producing bacteria. As these bacteria ferment glycogen into glucose and eventually lactic acid,[56,57] the resulting lowered pH is thought to establish an inhospitable environment that is critical in preventing the propagation of many bacterial taxa, including many pathogenic or less-healthy species. Traditionally, the high prevalence of lactic acid–producing bacteria has been considered the hallmark of vaginal health,[9] and, for many women, species of the genus *Lactobacillus* predominate the vaginal microbiome during the reproductive years.[58] As women approach menopause, estrogen levels decrease, glycogen content in the vaginal epithelium diminishes, and, as a result, lactobacilli decrease in prevalence.[59] With fewer lactobacilli present, less lactic acid is produced, and the vaginal pH increases. Hormone replacement therapy during and after menopause reverses this effect by increasing the glycogen content in the vaginal environment, which, in turn, has been reported to increase the predominance of *Lactobacillus* and significantly lower vaginal pH compared with postmenopausal women not undergoing hormone replacement therapy.[59–61]

The composition of vaginal bacterial communities differs dramatically among reproductive-age women of different ethnic groups.[12–14] Ravel and colleagues[12] analyzed the samples from 396 asymptomatic women and identified 5 community clusters: those predominated by *L iners*, *L crispatus*, *L gasseri*, or *L jensenii* or those that had low proportions of lactobacilli and high proportions of strictly anaerobic bacteria. They found that 80% to 90% of the bacterial communities characterized in Asian (n = 97) and white (n = 98) women were dominated by species of *Lactobacillus*. In contrast, only about 60% of Hispanic (n = 97) and African American (n = 104) women had vaginal microbiomes dominated by *Lactobacilli*. This compositional difference was reflected in the higher average pH values (ie, pH >4.5) recorded in Hispanic and African American women, which are above the range generally associated with vaginal health. A more extensive study by Fettweis and colleagues[14] of vaginal samples from 1686 African American women and 482 women of European ancestry showed similar results. However, in the latter study, two additional community clusters dominated by *G vaginalis* or BVAB1 were observed, and a significant number of the samples, predominantly those from African American women, did not cluster into a common profile (**Fig. 1**). Collectively, these findings show that the vaginal microbiome is much more heterogeneous and dynamic than commonly believed.

Although the influence of genetic factors on the vaginal microbiome is generally not well understood, a handful of genetic variants that impact vaginal health have been uncovered. The innate immune response in the female genital tract, which represents a pivotal defense against invading pathogens, represents one such genetically driven influence. On recognition of pathogen-associated molecular patterns through interaction with toll-like receptors, the innate immune response triggers secretion of a wide range of inflammatory mediators, chemokines and cytokines. Single nucleotide polymorphisms that disrupt proteins that mediate normal signaling or immune recognition have been associated with increased susceptibility to vaginal infections.[2,62,63] Moreover, polymorphisms in toll-like receptor-4, tumor necrosis factor–α, interleukin (IL)-4 and IL-10 genes have been found to induce aberrant responses to bacterial vaginosis (BV)-associated bacteria related to PTB.[62,64,65] Clearly, further investigation

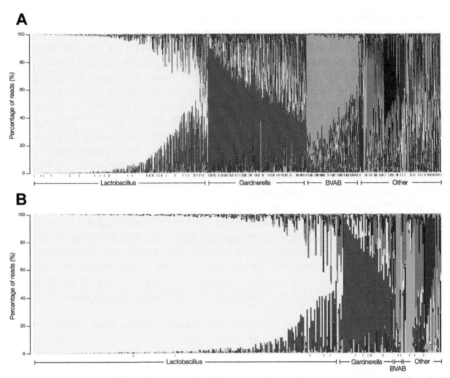

Fig. 1. Microbiome profiles of women of African American or European ancestry. Midvaginal relative abundance profiles using genus-level classification from (*A*) 960 African American women and (*B*) 330 women of European ancestry enrolled in the Vaginal Human Microbiome Project at VCU. The profiles are clustered by the dominant genus into different community types. All processed samples were represented by greater than 5000 reads. See Fettweis and colleagues[14] for methodology. Black vertical dashes represent women with a clinical BV diagnosis. (*Data from* Fettweis JM, Brooks JP, Serrano MG, et al. Differences in vaginal microbiome in African American women vs women of European ancestry. Microbiology 2014. [Epub ahead of print].)

into the impact of environmental and genetic influences on the vaginal microbiome have a strong potential to improve diagnostics and contribute to the development of more personalized medicine relevant to urogenital health of women.

THE VAGINAL MICROBIOME AND DISEASE

The dynamic equilibrium of the vaginal microbiome can be altered by environmental factors and external interferences (eg, antibiotics, vaginal hygiene, sexual intercourse, hormone therapy). These alterations can result in microbial imbalances or dysbiosis in the urogenital tract. As outlined above, the normally commensal bacterial communities present in the vagina can, under certain circumstances, become pathogenic (eg, *G vaginalis*, *E coli* and *C albicans*) if a shift in the equilibrium favors their competitiveness. Thus, changes in the vaginal microbiome can lead to intervals of increased susceptibility that negatively impact the ability of the community to resist pathogen colonization.

BACTERIAL VAGINOSIS

BV is a polymicrobial disorder and the most common vaginal imbalance in reproductive-age women worldwide, affecting between 20% and 25% of the general population and up to 50% of women visiting sexual health clinics.[66,67] Although normally treatable with antibiotics, recurrence is the norm. Thus, BV represents a significant public health challenge that predisposes affected women to sexually transmitted infections, pelvic inflammatory disease and numerous adverse pregnancy outcomes such as preterm birth and stillbirth.[68–70] Although it remains uncertain whether BV can be sexually transmitted, studies have found that BV increases the risk of transmission of HIV and other sexually transmitted diseases.[71,72] Although BV is not attributable to infection by a single pathogenic organism, multiple factors have been identified, including, but not limited to, a new sexual partner, douching, smoking and unsafe sexual practices that increase a woman's risk for BV. Relapsing BV is a major problem for many women, with recurrence rates greater than 50% within 12 months of treatment.[73]

Although its etiology is not well understood, and the disorder itself is rather loosely defined, BV is generally considered to be characterized by the disruption of the normal vaginal ecosystem marked by depletion of lactobacilli and overgrowth of various gram-negative or anaerobic bacteria, including G vaginalis, Atopobium vaginae, Megasphaera phylotype 1 species, Mobiluncus spp, Ureaplasma urealyticum, Prevotella, Peptostreptococcus and Mycoplasma hominis.[74,75] Although BV is considered a polymicrobial disease, G vaginalis has been promoted as an important contributor in the pathogenesis of BV and is present in 95% of cases.[76] G vaginalis adheres to and establishes a biofilm on the vaginal epithelium and secretes a cytotoxin that has the potential to disrupt and kill epithelial cells.[76] The massive increase of vaginal anaerobes in BV is associated with heightened production of proteolytic enzymes and the subsequent breakdown of vaginal peptides to a variety of amines. In high pH environments, the amines become malodorous, contribute to the typical vaginal discharge and trigger the release of proinflammatory cytokines such as IL-1β and IL-8.[77,78] Women with BV typically complain of vaginal discharge and a fishy malodor. However, a substantial fraction of women with bacterial populations characteristic of BV are asymptomatic and report no clinical complaints.

BV is typically diagnosed based on the presence of three of the following Amsel criteria[79]: (1) an elevated vaginal pH level (>4.5); (2) a thin, homogeneous gray-white discharge; (3) a fishy odor upon the addition of 10% potassium hydroxide to vaginal fluid on a glass slide; and (4) presence of clue cells (squamous epithelial cells covered with adherent bacteria) on microscopic examination of vaginal fluid. Alternatively, in research and laboratory settings, BV is diagnosed by scoring a gram-stained vaginal smear using the Nugent criteria.[80] The Nugent score assumes high numbers of Lactobacillus species indicate health, and their depletion coupled with increased numbers of small or curved gram-variable rods indicates BV.

It is well established that there is a greater incidence of BV among African American women. Fettweis and colleagues[14] compared the microbiome profiles of African American women and women of European ancestry with and without a clinical diagnosis of BV (see **Fig. 1**). Of the healthy subjects, those who did not receive a clinical diagnosis, African American women (n = 728) were more likely to be colonized by strict anaerobes, whereas women of European ancestry were more likely colonized by L crispatus, L gasseri and L jensenii. Furthermore, of the participants with a positive diagnosis for BV, African American women (n = 373) were more likely colonized by Anaerococcus tetradius, BVAB1 and BVAB3, Coriobacteriaceae, Sneathia species,

Parvimonas, Dialister, Megasphaera, Bulleidia, Prevotella species and *A vaginae*, whereas women of European ancestry were more likely colonized by *M hominis*, *Dialister micraerophilus* and an undefined *Gemella* species. This study extends previous findings[16,57] that, even among apparently healthy women, African American ethnicity is associated with a vaginal microbiome that more closely resembles BV, characterized by an increase in species diversity and decrease in lactobacilli (see **Fig. 1**). As of yet, the basis for this disparity remains unclear. The increased risk of BV among African American women parallels their increased risk for PTB, and a cause-and-effect relationship is sometimes inferred. However, the role of this microbial diversity in adverse outcomes in pregnancy remains unproven, and a better understanding of the factors associated with ethnicity that contribute to the vaginal microbiome has important implications for reproductive health.

Several vaginal species (eg, *L iners*, *P bivia*, and *A vaginae*) have been detected in vaginal samples from healthy women and from women with BV, indicating that these species have evolved mechanisms to persist in vastly differing environments. Among the vaginal lactobacilli, *L iners* is unique in its ability to survive in a BV-like environment. In a recent study, Macklaim and colleagues[81] used RNA-seq strategies to describe the difference in gene expression profiles of *L iners* isolated from healthy women and women with BV environments.[81,82] These studies showed that *L iners* upregulates expression of a cholesterol-dependent cytolysin (CDC) in a woman with BV. CDCs belong to a family of pore-forming toxins that are common to many pathogenic bacteria, including *G vaginalis*, but absent in *L crispatus*, *L jensenii*, or *L gasseri*. The *L iners*–encoded CDC exhibits 55% amino acid identity to the vaginolysin of *G vaginalis*, which is thought to induce epithelial cell cytotoxicity.[83,84] In contrast to the lactic acid–rich environment of the classical healthy vagina, the dominant metabolic byproducts of *L iners* in the vagina of a woman with BV include succinate and a panel of short-chain fatty acids. Relevant to BV, increased production of succinate supports the growth of anaerobic bacteria. This study[81] shows the ability of *L iners* to regulate gene expression depending on environmental factors (ie, bacterial composition, pH level) and highlights the need for metatranscriptomic analyses to fully resolve species-specific interactions in the context of the host and community.

Although *A vaginae* has been associated with both healthy, asymptomatic women and women with BV, there has been debate over whether this lactic acid–producing species is a common component of the vaginal microbiota. A recent study using in vitro colonization of vaginal epithelial cell monolayers with *L crispatus*, *L iners*, *P bivia* and *A vaginae* found that each species triggers a unique innate immune signature.[2] Consistent with the apparently beneficial role of *L crispatus*, exposure of this bacterium to epithelial cells resulted in low-level immune activation. Alternatively, *A vaginae* elicited a robust inflammatory response and increased expression of mucin-encoding genes.[2] Furthermore, studies have reported an association between increased levels of *A vaginae* and *G vaginalis* with preterm labor.[85]

PREGNANCY AND PRETERM BIRTH

The vaginal microbiome changes during pregnancy, growing increasingly homogeneous as pregnancy progresses.[86,87] A recent longitudinal study by Romero and colleagues[87] analyzed the taxonomic 16S rRNA profiles of vaginal samples from 22 pregnant and 32 nonpregnant women to investigate the temporal dynamics of the vaginal microbiota stability throughout pregnancy. They reported that the microbial communities of nonpregnant women sometimes undergo regular shifts in the representation and abundance of *Lactobacillus* species. In contrast, throughout pregnancy, the vaginal microbiota is normally dominated by *Lactobacillus* species.

PTB, defined as a birth before 37 weeks of gestation, affects more than 11.5% of births and contributes to more than one-third of all infant deaths.[88,89] Very PTBs (<32 weeks) are commonly the result of infection in the uterine cavity caused by ascension of vaginal bacteria through the cervix.[90] The most prevalent species associated with PTB are *U urealyticum, M hominis, Bacteroides* spp., *G. vaginalis* and *Fusobacterium nucleatum*.[90,91] Bacteria identified in PTB-associated infections have been detected in umbilical cord blood, amniotic fluid, fetal membranes and placenta.[90] However, infection of the uterine cavity does not always lead to adverse outcome, and studies suggest that inflammation plays a more direct role in PTB.[92]

It is well established that diagnosed BV is associated with an increased risk for PTB, but the most prominent risk factor for PTB is a previous PTB.[93] As outlined above, this observation is also consistent with the fact that BV is a recurrent if not chronic problem for many women. A recent study reported that, among women with a history of PTB, women with high levels of *Sneathia* species, BVAB1 and *Mobiluncus* species early in pregnancy were significantly more likely to experience a spontaneous PTB.[94] We recently reported that the genome of a *Sneathia amnii* strain from a woman who experienced preterm birth bears various potential pathogenic determinants including cytotoxins and adhesins. We also found that *S amnii* forms pores in and kills eukaryotic cells in culture.[36] Continued identification and study of bacteria with strong predictive value holds promise for developing more effective prophylactic and therapeutic approaches to reduce rates of PTB.

SUMMARY

Although not as diverse as the gut or oral microbiomes, deep sequence analysis of the vaginal microbiome is revealing an unexpected complexity that was not anticipated as recently as several years ago. Studies have found that women can be clustered into a finite number of groups based on the profile and complexity of their microbiomes. Some of these groups are diverse and comprise complex combinations of bacterial taxa. Defying convention, even apparently healthy women often display these complex microbiome profiles. Conversely, many women with BV exhibit homogenous vaginal microbiomes dominated by lactobacilli, underscoring the likely multiple etiologies of the syndrome of BV, and calling for more diagnostic accuracy and resolution. African American women have more diverse microbiomes, more BV, and more PTB than women of European ancestry. However, the lack of clarity in the definition of a healthy vaginal microbiome, much less an unhealthy vaginal microbiome, underscores the need for more investigation of these phenomena. Some clarity may be gained by the careful analysis of the genomes of the specific bacteria in these women. We know that bacteria with identical 16S rRNA sequences (eg, the many strains of *E coli*) have vastly different pathogenic potentials. Thus, it may not be surprising that one healthy woman's vaginal microbiome is dominated by *G vaginalis* with an identical 16S rRNA signature to that of a *G vaginalis* strain populating the vagina of a woman with BV or other unhealthy condition. Ongoing studies will clarify this process and offer relief for women with recurring vaginal maladies and hope for pregnant women to avoid the experience of PTB.

ACKNOWLEDGMENTS

The authors thank members of the Vaginal Microbiome Consortium (vmc.vcu.edu) at VCU for their effort and inspiration in generation of the data and its analysis associated with this publication. Sequence analysis was performed in the Nucleic Acids Research Facilities at VCU. Bioinformatics analysis was provided by the staff of the Bioinformatics Computational Core Laboratories at VCU.

REFERENCES

1. Cash HL, Whitham CV, Behrendt CL, et al. Symbiotic bacteria direct expression of an intestinal bactericidal lectin. Science 2006;313(5790):1126–30. http://dx.doi.org/10.1126/science.1127119.
2. Doerflinger SY, Throop AL, Herbst-Kralovetz MM. Bacteria in the vaginal microbiome alter the innate immune response and barrier properties of the human vaginal epithelia in a species-specific manner. J Infect Dis 2014. http://dx.doi.org/10.1093/infdis/jiu004.
3. NIH HMP Working Group, Peterson J, Garges S, et al. The NIH Human Microbiome Project. Genome Res 2009;19(12):2317–23. http://dx.doi.org/10.1101/gr.096651.109.
4. Ehrlich S. MetaHIT: the european union project on metagenomics of the human intestinal tract. In: Nelson KE, editor. Metagenomics of the human body. New York: Springer; 2011. p. 307–16. http://dx.doi.org/10.1007/978-1-4419-7089-3_15.
5. Arumugam M, Raes J, Pelletier E, et al. Enterotypes of the human gut microbiome. Nature 2011;473(7346):174–80. http://dx.doi.org/10.1038/nature09944.
6. Anderson LS, Beverly WT, Corey LA, et al. The mid-atlantic twin registry. Twin Res 2002;5(5):449–55. http://dx.doi.org/10.1375/136905202320906264.
7. Kuczynski J, Lauber CL, Walters WA, et al. Experimental and analytical tools for studying the human microbiome. Nat Rev Genet 2012;13(1):47–58. http://dx.doi.org/10.1038/nrg3129.
8. Fettweis JM, Serrano MG, Sheth NU, et al. Species-level classification of the vaginal microbiome. BMC Genomics 2012;13(Suppl 8):S17. http://dx.doi.org/10.1186/1471-2164-13-S8-S17.
9. Donders GG, Bosmans E, Dekeersmaecker A, et al. Pathogenesis of abnormal vaginal bacterial flora. Am J Obstet Gynecol 2000;182(4):872–8.
10. Aroutcheva A, Gariti D, Simon M, et al. Defense factors of vaginal lactobacilli. Am J Obstet Gynecol 2001;185(2):375–9. http://dx.doi.org/10.1067/mob.2001.115867.
11. Eschenbach DA, Davick PR, Williams BL, et al. Prevalence of hydrogen peroxide-producing lactobacillus species in normal women and women with bacterial vaginosis. J Clin Microbiol 1989;27(2):251–6.
12. Ravel J, Gajer P, Abdo Z, et al. Vaginal microbiome of reproductive-age women. Proc Natl Acad Sci U S A 2011;108(Suppl 1):4680–7.
13. Yamamoto T, Zhou X, Williams CJ, et al. Bacterial populations in the vaginas of healthy adolescent women. J Pediatr Adolesc Gynecol 2009;22(1):11–8.
14. Fettweis JM, Brooks JP, Serrano MG, et al. Differences in vaginal microbiome in african american women versus women of european ancestry. Microbiology 2014. http://dx.doi.org/10.1099/mic.0.081034-0.
15. Pavlova SI, Kilic AO, Kilic SS, et al. Genetic diversity of vaginal lactobacilli from women in different countries based on 16S rRNA gene sequences. J Appl Microbiol 2002;92(3):451–9.
16. Zhou X, Bent SJ, Schneider MG, et al. Characterization of vaginal microbial communities in adult healthy women using cultivation-independent methods. Microbiology 2004;150(Pt 8):2565–73.

17. Gajer P, Brotman RM, Bai G, et al. Temporal dynamics of the human vaginal microbiota. Sci Transl Med 2012;4(132):132ra52. http://dx.doi.org/10.1126/scitranslmed.3003605.

18. Witkin SS, Mendes-Soares H, Linhares IM, et al. Influence of vaginal bacteria and d- and l-lactic acid isomers on vaginal extracellular matrix metalloproteinase inducer: implications for protection against upper genital tract infections. MBio 2013;4(4). http://dx.doi.org/10.1128/mBio.00460-13.

19. O'Hanlon DE, Moench TR, Cone RA. Vaginal pH and microbicidal lactic acid when lactobacilli dominate the microbiota. PLoS One 2013;8(11):e80074. http://dx.doi.org/10.1371/journal.pone.0080074.

20. O'Hanlon DE, Moench TR, Cone RA. In vaginal fluid, bacteria associated with bacterial vaginosis can be suppressed with lactic acid but not hydrogen peroxide. BMC Infect Dis 2011;11:200. http://dx.doi.org/10.1186/1471-2334-11-200.

21. O'Hanlon DE, Lanier BR, Moench TR, et al. Cervicovaginal fluid and semen block the microbicidal activity of hydrogen peroxide produced by vaginal lactobacilli. BMC Infect Dis 2010;10:120. http://dx.doi.org/10.1186/1471-2334-10-120.

22. Selle K, Klaenhammer TR. Genomic and phenotypic evidence for probiotic influences of lactobacillus gasseri on human health. FEMS Microbiol Rev 2013; 37(6):915–35. http://dx.doi.org/10.1111/1574-6976.12021.

23. Zárate G, Nader-Macias ME. Influence of probiotic vaginal lactobacilli on in vitro adhesion of urogenital pathogens to vaginal epithelial cells. Lett Appl Microbiol 2006;43(2):174–80. http://dx.doi.org/10.1111/j.1472-765X.2006.01934.x.

24. Zárate G, Santos V, Nader-Macias ME. Protective effect of vaginal lactobacillus paracasei cRL 1289 against urogenital infection produced by staphylococcus aureus in a mouse animal model. Infect Dis Obstet Gynecol 2009;2009:48358. http://dx.doi.org/10.1155/2007/48358.

25. Boris S, Suárez JE, Vázquez F, et al. Adherence of human vaginal lactobacilli to vaginal epithelial cells and interaction with uropathogens. Infect Immun 1998; 66(5):1985–9.

26. O'Sullivan O, O'Callaghan J, Sangrador-Vegas A, et al. Comparative genomics of lactic acid bacteria reveals a niche-specific gene set. BMC Microbiol 2009;9: 50. http://dx.doi.org/10.1186/1471-2180-9-50.

27. Mendes-Soares H, Suzuki H, Hickey RJ, et al. Comparative functional genomics of lactobacillus spp. reveals possible mechanisms for specialization of vaginal lactobacilli to their environment. J Bacteriol 2014. http://dx.doi.org/10.1128/JB.01439-13.

28. Atassi F, Brassart D, Grob P, et al. Lactobacillus strains isolated from the vaginal microbiota of healthy women inhibit prevotella bivia and gardnerella vaginalis in coculture and cell culture. FEMS Immunol Med Microbiol 2006;48(3):424–32. http://dx.doi.org/10.1111/j.1574-695X.2006.00162.x.

29. Kaewsrichan J, Peeyananjarassri K, Kongprasertkit J. Selection and identification of anaerobic lactobacilli producing inhibitory compounds against vaginal pathogens. FEMS Immunol Med Microbiol 2006;48(1):75–83. http://dx.doi.org/10.1111/j.1574-695X.2006.00124.x.

30. Osset J, Bartolomé RM, García E, et al. Assessment of the capacity of lactobacillus to inhibit the growth of uropathogens and block their adhesion to vaginal epithelial cells. J Infect Dis 2001;183(3):485–91. http://dx.doi.org/10.1086/318070.

31. Spurbeck RR, Arvidson CG. Inhibition of neisseria gonorrhoeae epithelial cell interactions by vaginal lactobacillus species. Infect Immun 2008;76(7):3124–30. http://dx.doi.org/10.1128/IAI.00101-08.

32. Mastromarino P, Brigidi P, Macchia S, et al. Characterization and selection of vaginal lactobacillus strains for the preparation of vaginal tablets. J Appl Microbiol 2002;93(5):884–93.

33. Reid G, McGroarty JA, Angotti R, et al. Lactobacillus inhibitor production against escherichia coli and coaggregation ability with uropathogens. Can J Microbiol 1988;34(3):344–51.

34. Hyman RW, Fukushima M, Diamond L, et al. Microbes on the human vaginal epithelium. Proc Natl Acad Sci U S A 2005;102(22):7952–7. http://dx.doi.org/10.1073/pnas.0503236102.

35. Verhelst R, Verstraelen H, Claeys G, et al. Cloning of 16S rRNA genes amplified from normal and disturbed vaginal microflora suggests a strong association between Atopobium vaginae, Gardnerella vaginalis and bacterial vaginosis. BMC Microbiol 2004;4:16.

36. Harwich MD Jr, Serrano MG, Fettweis JM, et al. Genomic sequence analysis and characterization of sneathia amnii sp. nov. BMC Genomics 2012;13(Suppl 8):S4. http://dx.doi.org/10.1186/1471-2164-13-S8-S4.

37. Shi Y, Chen L, Tong J, et al. Preliminary characterization of vaginal microbiota in healthy chinese women using cultivation-independent methods. J Obstet Gynaecol Res 2009;35(3):525–32. http://dx.doi.org/10.1111/j.1447-0756.2008.00971.x.

38. Witkin SS, Ledger WJ. Complexities of the uniquely human vagina. Sci Transl Med 2012;4(132):132fs11. http://dx.doi.org/10.1126/scitranslmed.3003944.

39. Johnson SR, Petzold CR, Galask RP. Qualitative and quantitative changes of the vaginal microbial flora during the menstrual cycle. Am J Reprod Immunol Microbiol 1985;9(1):1–5.

40. Eschenbach DA, Thwin SS, Patton DL, et al. Influence of the normal menstrual cycle on vaginal tissue, discharge, and microflora. Clin Infect Dis 2000;30(6):901–7.

41. Mitchell CM, Fredricks DN, Winer RL, et al. Effect of sexual debut on vaginal microbiota in a cohort of young women. Obstet Gynecol 2012;120(6):1306–13. http://dx.doi.org/10.1097/AOG.0b013e31827075ac.

42. Hooton TM, Fennell CL, Clark AM, et al. Nonoxynol-9: differential antibacterial activity and enhancement of bacterial adherence to vaginal epithelial cells. J Infect Dis 1991;164(6):1216–9.

43. Hooton TM, Hillier S, Johnson C, et al. Escherichia coli bacteriuria and contraceptive method. JAMA 1991;265(1):64–9.

44. Aagaard K, Ma J, Antony KM, et al. The placenta harbors a unique microbiome. Sci Transl Med 2014;6(237):237ra65. http://dx.doi.org/10.1126/scitranslmed.3008599.

45. Stout MJ, Conlon B, Landeau M, et al. Identification of intracellular bacteria in the basal plate of the human placenta in term and preterm gestations. Am J Obstet Gynecol 2013;208(3):226.e1–7. http://dx.doi.org/10.1016/j.ajog.2013.01.018.

46. Romero R, Schaudinn C, Kusanovic JP, et al. Detection of a microbial biofilm in intraamniotic infection. Am J Obstet Gynecol 2008;198(1):135.e1–5. http://dx.doi.org/10.1016/j.ajog.2007.11.026.

47. Mändar R, Mikelsaar M. Transmission of mother's microflora to the newborn at birth. Biol Neonate 1996;69(1):30–5.

48. Dominguez-Bello MG, Costello EK, Contreras M, et al. Delivery mode shapes the acquisition and structure of the initial microbiota across multiple body habitats in newborns. Proc Natl Acad Sci U S A 2010;107(26):11971–5.

49. Jiménez E, Marín ML, Martín R, et al. Is meconium from healthy newborns actually sterile? Res Microbiol 2008;159(3):187–93. http://dx.doi.org/10.1016/j.resmic.2007.12.007.

50. Ardissone AN, de la Cruz DM, Davis-Richardson AG, et al. Meconium microbiome analysis identifies bacteria correlated with premature birth. PLoS One 2014;9(3):e90784. http://dx.doi.org/10.1371/journal.pone.0090784.

51. Makino H, Kushiro A, Ishikawa E, et al. Transmission of intestinal bifidobacterium longum subsp. longum strains from mother to infant, determined by multilocus sequencing typing and amplified fragment length polymorphism. Appl Environ Microbiol 2011;77(19):6788–93. http://dx.doi.org/10.1128/AEM.05346-11.

52. Makino H, Kushiro A, Ishikawa E, et al. Mother-to-infant transmission of intestinal bifidobacterial strains has an impact on the early development of vaginally delivered infant's microbiota. PLoS One 2013;8(11):e78331. http://dx.doi.org/10.1371/journal.pone.0078331.

53. Hammerschlag MR, Alpert S, Rosner I, et al. Microbiology of the vagina in children: normal and potentially pathogenic organisms. Pediatrics 1978;62(1):57–62.

54. Hammerschlag MR, Alpert S, Onderdonk AB, et al. Anaerobic microflora of the vagina in children. Am J Obstet Gynecol 1978;131(8):853–6.

55. Jaquiery A, Stylianopoulos A, Hogg G, et al. Vulvovaginitis: clinical features, aetiology, and microbiology of the genital tract. Arch Dis Child 1999;81(1):64–7.

56. Paavonen J. Physiology and ecology of the vagina. Scand J Infect Dis Suppl 1983;40:31–5.

57. Zhou X, Brown CJ, Abdo Z, et al. Differences in the composition of vaginal microbial communities found in healthy Caucasian and black women. ISME J 2007;1(2):121–33.

58. Jennifer FA, Buck G. The vaginal microbiome: disease, genetics and the environment. 2011. Available at: http://dxdoiorg/101038/npre201151502.

59. Gupta S, Kumar N, Singhal N, et al. Vaginal microflora in postmenopausal women on hormone replacement therapy. Indian J Pathol Microbiol 2006;49(3):457–61.

60. Burton JP, Reid G. Evaluation of the bacterial vaginal flora of 20 postmenopausal women by direct (Nugent score) and molecular (polymerase chain reaction and denaturing gradient gel electrophoresis) techniques. J Infect Dis 2002;186(12):1770–80.

61. Pabich WL, Fihn SD, Stamm WE, et al. Prevalence and determinants of vaginal flora alterations in postmenopausal women. J Infect Dis 2003;188(7):1054–8. http://dx.doi.org/10.1086/378203.

62. Genc MR, Onderdonk A. Endogenous bacterial flora in pregnant women and the influence of maternal genetic variation. BJOG 2011;118(2):154–63. http://dx.doi.org/10.1111/j.1471-0528.2010.02772.x.

63. Verstraelen H, Verhelst R, Nuytinck L, et al. Gene polymorphisms of toll-like and related recognition receptors in relation to the vaginal carriage of gardnerella vaginalis and atopobium vaginae. J Reprod Immunol 2009;79(2):163–73. http://dx.doi.org/10.1016/j.jri.2008.10.006.

64. Genc MR, Schantz-Dunn J. The role of gene-environment interaction in predicting adverse pregnancy outcome. Best Pract Res Clin Obstet Gynaecol 2007;21(3):491–504. http://dx.doi.org/10.1016/j.bpobgyn.2007.01.009.

65. Jones NM, Holzman C, Friderici KH, et al. Interplay of cytokine polymorphisms and bacterial vaginosis in the etiology of preterm delivery. J Reprod Immunol 2010;87(1–2):82–9. http://dx.doi.org/10.1016/j.jri.2010.06.158.

66. Morris M, Nicoll A, Simms I, et al. Bacterial vaginosis: a public health review. BJOG 2001;108(5):439–50.
67. Srinivasan S, Fredricks DN. The human vaginal bacterial biota and bacterial vaginosis. Interdiscip Perspect Infect Dis 2008;2008:750479. http://dx.doi.org/10.1155/2008/750479.
68. Leitich H, Bodner-Adler B, Brunbauer M, et al. Bacterial vaginosis as a risk factor for preterm delivery: a meta-analysis. Am J Obstet Gynecol 2003;189(1):139–47.
69. Hillier SL, Krohn MA, Cassen E, et al. The role of bacterial vaginosis and vaginal bacteria in amniotic fluid infection in women in preterm labor with intact fetal membranes. Clin Infect Dis 1995;20(Suppl 2):S276–8.
70. Sweet RL. Role of bacterial vaginosis in pelvic inflammatory disease. Clin Infect Dis 1995;20(Suppl 2):S271–5.
71. Schmid G, Markowitz L, Joesoef R, et al. Bacterial vaginosis and HIV infection. Sex Transm Infect 2000;76(1):3–4.
72. Wiesenfeld HC, Hillier SL, Krohn MA, et al. Bacterial vaginosis is a strong predictor of neisseria gonorrhoeae and chlamydia trachomatis infection. Clin Infect Dis 2003;36(5):663–8. http://dx.doi.org/10.1086/367658.
73. Bradshaw CS, Morton AN, Hocking J, et al. High recurrence rates of bacterial vaginosis over the course of 12 months after oral metronidazole therapy and factors associated with recurrence. J Infect Dis 2006;193(11):1478–86. http://dx.doi.org/10.1086/503780.
74. Fredricks DN, Fiedler TL, Marrazzo JM. Molecular identification of bacteria associated with bacterial vaginosis. N Engl J Med 2005;353(18):1899–911.
75. Swidsinski A, Mendling W, Loening-Baucke V, et al. Adherent biofilms in bacterial vaginosis. Obstet Gynecol 2005;106(5 Pt 1):1013–23. http://dx.doi.org/10.1097/01.AOG.0000183594.45524.d2.
76. Patterson JL, Stull-Lane A, Girerd PH, et al. Analysis of adherence, biofilm formation and cytotoxicity suggests a greater virulence potential of gardnerella vaginalis relative to other bacterial-vaginosis-associated anaerobes. Microbiology 2010;156(Pt 2):392–9. http://dx.doi.org/10.1099/mic.0.034280-0.
77. Hedges SR, Barrientes F, Desmond RA, et al. Local and systemic cytokine levels in relation to changes in vaginal flora. J Infect Dis 2006;193(4):556–62. http://dx.doi.org/10.1086/499824.
78. Beigi RH, Yudin MH, Cosentino L, et al. Cytokines, pregnancy, and bacterial vaginosis: comparison of levels of cervical cytokines in pregnant and nonpregnant women with bacterial vaginosis. J Infect Dis 2007;196(9):1355–60. http://dx.doi.org/10.1086/521628.
79. Amsel R, Totten PA, Spiegel CA, et al. Nonspecific vaginitis. Diagnostic criteria and microbial and epidemiologic associations. Am J Med 1983;74(1):14–22.
80. Nugent RP, Krohn MA, Hillier SL. Reliability of diagnosing bacterial vaginosis is improved by a standardized method of gram stain interpretation. J Clin Microbiol 1991;29(2):297–301.
81. Macklaim JM, Fernandes AD, Di Bella JM, et al. Comparative meta-RNA-seq of the vaginal microbiota and differential expression by Lactobacillus iners in health and dysbiosis. Microbiome 2013;1:12.
82. Zozaya-Hinchliffe M, Lillis R, Martin DH, et al. Quantitative pCR assessments of bacterial species in women with and without bacterial vaginosis. J Clin Microbiol 2010;48(5):1812–9. http://dx.doi.org/10.1128/JCM.00851-09.
83. Randis TM, Zaklama J, LaRocca TJ, et al. Vaginolysin drives epithelial ultrastructural responses to gardnerella vaginalis. Infect Immun 2013;81(12):4544–50. http://dx.doi.org/10.1128/IAI.00627-13.

84. Macklaim JM, Gloor GB, Anukam KC, et al. At the crossroads of vaginal health and disease, the genome sequence of lactobacillus iners aB-1. Proc Natl Acad Sci U S A 2011;108(Suppl 1):4688–95. http://dx.doi.org/10.1073/pnas.1000086107.

85. Menard J-P, Fenollar F, Henry M, et al. Molecular quantification of gardnerella vaginalis and atopobium vaginae loads to predict bacterial vaginosis. Clin Infect Dis 2008;47(1):33–43. http://dx.doi.org/10.1086/588661.

86. Aagaard K, Riehle K, Ma J, et al. A metagenomic approach to characterization of the vaginal microbiome signature in pregnancy. PLoS One 2012;7(6):e36466. http://dx.doi.org/10.1371/journal.pone.0036466.

87. Romero R, Hassan SS, Gajer P, et al. The composition and stability of the vaginal microbiota of normal pregnant women is different from that of non-pregnant women. Microbiome 2014;2(1):4. http://dx.doi.org/10.1186/2049-2618-2-4.

88. Goldenberg RL, Culhane JF, Iams JD, et al. Epidemiology and causes of pre-term birth. Lancet 2008;371(9606):75–84. http://dx.doi.org/10.1016/S0140-6736(08)60074-4.

89. Iacovidou N, Varsami M, Syggellou A. Neonatal outcome of preterm delivery. Ann N Y Acad Sci 2010;1205:130–4.

90. Goldenberg RL, Hauth JC, Andrews WW. Intrauterine infection and preterm delivery. N Engl J Med 2000;342(20):1500–7. http://dx.doi.org/10.1056/NEJM200005183422007.

91. Jefferson KK. The bacterial etiology of preterm birth. Adv Appl Microbiol 2012;80:1–22. http://dx.doi.org/10.1016/B978-0-12-394381-1.00001-5.

92. Combs CA, Gravett M, Garite TJ, et al. Amniotic fluid infection, inflammation, and colonization in preterm labor with intact membranes. Am J Obstet Gynecol 2014;210(2):125.e1–15. http://dx.doi.org/10.1016/j.ajog.2013.11.032.

93. Mercer BM, Goldenberg RL, Moawad AH, et al. The preterm prediction study: effect of gestational age and cause of preterm birth on subsequent obstetric outcome. National institute of child health and human development maternal-fetal medicine units network. Am J Obstet Gynecol 1999;181(5 Pt 1):1216–21.

94. Nelson DB, Hanlon A, Nachamkin I, et al. Early pregnancy changes in bacterial vaginosis-associated bacteria and preterm delivery. Paediatr Perinat Epidemiol 2014. http://dx.doi.org/10.1111/ppe.12106.

The Genetic Predisposition and the Interplay of Host Genetics and Gut Microbiome in Crohn Disease

 CrossMark

Hu Jianzhong, PhD

KEYWORDS

- Gut microbiome • Host genetics • Crohn disease

KEY POINTS

- Association between host genetics and Crohn disease.
- Association between gut microbiome and Crohn disease.
- Effect of Crohn disease–associated host genetics on gut microbiome.

HOST GENETICS AND CROHN DISEASE

Crohn disease (CD) is an inflammatory bowel disease (IBD) resulting from defects in the regulatory constraints on mucosal immune response to enteric bacteria, which arises in genetically predisposed individuals.[1,2] Common manifestations of CD include inflammation, diarrhea, and weight loss. According to a report by the US Centers for Disease Control and Prevention, CD may affect more than 700,000 individuals in the United States alone. Geographic statistics showed that the incidence and prevalence of CD also increase across time and in other countries around the world, indicating its emergence as a global disease.[3–5] CD has no gender preference and can occur at any age, but it is more prevalent among adolescents and young adults between the ages of 15 and 35 years.[6] Extensive genetic studies involving linkage analyses, candidate gene studies, and, most recently, genome-wide association studies (GWAS) with imputation and meta-analyses to combine the power of multiple individual GWAS have identified more than 140 loci predisposing to CD.[1,7,8] Emerging evidence from network analysis and biological function studies has shown that many major CD susceptibility loci encode genes involved in cross-talked complex pathways of host

The authors declare that there are no conflicts of interest.
Department of Genetics and Genomic Sciences, Icahn School of Medicine at Mount Sinai, 1425 Madison Avenue, 14-70 Icahn Building, New York, NY 10029, USA
E-mail address: Jianzhong.hu@mssm.edu

Clin Lab Med 34 (2014) 763–770
http://dx.doi.org/10.1016/j.cll.2014.08.003
0272-2712/14/$ – see front matter © 2014 Elsevier Inc. All rights reserved.

labmed.theclinics.com

immune responses. Jostins and colleagues[8] further grouped these genes into several major immunologic pathways, including:

- Genes involved in T-cell circulating, including many specific T-cell subsets, such as T-helper cells (TH17 cells) (*STAT3*), memory T cells (*SP110*), and regulatory T cells (*STAT5B*).
- Genes in recognition of microbial-associated molecular patterns, including bacterial or fungi sensors *NOD1*,[9] *CARD9*, *NOD2/CARD15*,[10–17] and toll-like receptors (*TLRs*).
- Genes involved in autophagy process, including *IRGM*, encoding an autophagy protein that plays an important role in innate immunity against intracellular pathogens and CD-associated adherent-invasive *Escherichia coli* bacteria[18–20]; *ATG16L1*, a key component of the autophagy complex that processes and kills intracellular microbes,[11,13,17,21] and *LRRK2*, encoding a complex protein with multiple functional domains, recently found to regulate autophagosome formation through a calcium-dependent pathway.[22]
- Genes involved in maintenance of epithelial barrier integrity, including *DLG5*, encoding a member of the family of disks large (DLG) homologs with proposed function in the transmission of extracellular signals to the cytoskeleton and in the maintenance of epithelial cell structure[23]; fucosyltransferase 2 (*FUT2*) encoding an enzyme to synthesize the H antigen in body fluids and on the intestinal mucosa. A recent study suggested its role in CD pathogenesis by reprogramming the gut microbiome energy metabolism[24]; and other genes, including *BPI*, *DMBT1*, *IBD5*, *ITLN1*, *MUC1*, *MUC19*, *NKX2-3*, *SLC22A5*, *PTGER4*, *XBP1*, *ZNF365*.[8]
- Genes in regulation of cytokine production, specifically interferon-γ, interleukin 12 (IL-12), tumor necrosis factor α, IL-10 signaling, *IL17*, *IL18RAP*, *CCR6*, and so forth.
- Genes with proposed function in other immunologic processes.

MICROBIOME AND CROHN DISEASE

Although CD has a strong genetic predisposition, overall, only ∼14% total phenotypic variances of CD can be explained by risk loci.[8] Epidemiologic studies suggest that environmental factors are also essential contributors to the CD pathogenesis. For instance, smoking has been shown to be a risk factor for CD.[25] Many other environmental factors for IBD, including diet, infectious agents, medicine, stress, and social factors have been investigated. Those environmental factors may act independently or synergistically with genetic factors on the CD pathogenesis.

Recently, many studies have found that the identity and relative abundance of members of human-associated microbial communities are associated with different states of CD.[26,27] Microbes that live on and inside the human body (microbiota) consist of more than 100 trillion microbial cells and outnumber the quantity of the host cells by a factor of 10:1.[28] Commensal bacteria provide a wide range of metabolic functions that the human body lacks. They facilitate diverse processes such as digestion, absorption, and storage of nutrients, as well as protection against pathogen colonization through competition for nutrients, secretion of antimicrobial substances, and microniche exclusion.[29] Commensal bacteria also promote angiogenesis and development of the intestinal epithelium and have been shown to be essential for the normal development and function of the immune system.[29] Although miniscule inoculations of particular pathogenic strains can cause disease, little is known about whether there are core microbiome profiles that we all share in health and disease.[30–35] Although more studies on unrelated healthy adults have shown substantial diversity in their gut communities, the sampling sizes are often moderate, and how this diversity is affected by the host genetics or relates to function remains obscure.

Distinctive membership and composition of the gut microbiota have been shown to play a significant role in CD pathogenesis.[32,36,37] One recent study of 231 patients with IBD and healthy control individuals[38] showed that microbiome profiles are different between patients with CD and healthy control individuals. Particularly, compared with the healthy controls, the abundance of *Roseburia*, *Phascolarctobacterium*, Ruminococcaceae, and *Faecalibacterium* were reduced and *Clostridium* and *Escherichia/Shigella* were enriched in patients with CD. Some differences were observed only in tissue biopsies but not fecal samples. Another recent study of 447 pediatric patients with CD and 221 control individuals[39] showed that enrichment in Enterobacteriaceae, Pasteurellacaea, Veillonellaceae, and Fusobacteriaceae, and depletion in Erysipelotrichales, Bacteroidales, and Clostridiales, correlates strongly with disease status. This microbiome study also suggested that antibiotic exposure might amplify the microbial dysbiosis associated with CD.

EFFECT OF CROHN DISEASE–ASSOCIATED HOST GENETICS ON GUT MICROBIOME

Because many CD-associated host genes are related to microbial recognition, response, and clearance, it is expected that the variation on those genes may substantially affect the composition or structure of the gut microbiome. Many studies using host candidate gene deletions in animal models have observed associated substantial changes in microbiota. Although few human studies have elucidated the role of host genotype in reshaping the microbiota composition, a recent study of pediatric patients with CD[40] reported the covariations between the host ileal gene expression and the ileal microbiome communities, suggesting a global link between the host genetics and microbiome. Several major CD susceptibility genes have been reported to modulate the gut microbiome. Those genes are involved in 3 host immune pathways.

Recognition of Microbial-Associated Molecular Patterns

NOD2/CARD15 gene is one of the major susceptibility genes for CD.[14,16] Its gene product detects bacterial peptidoglycan found in both gram-positive and gram-negative bacteria and stimulates the host innate immune response. Several animal studies[41–43] reported that the deficiency of *NOD2* in mice resulted in substantially altered gut microbiome composition. At phylum level, the abundance of both ileal-associated and fecal-associated Bacteroidaceae was significantly increased in *NOD2*-deficient mice compared with wild-type mice.[41,42,44] In addition, the overall bacterial loads in the feces and terminal ileum of *NOD2*-deficient mice were significantly increased.[42] This finding might be partly explained because *NOD2* regulate the expression of antimicrobial peptide β-defensin-2.[45] In addition, the *NOD2* gene expression is inducible by the presence of commensal bacteria,[41] suggesting a possible feedback loop in regulating *NOD2* expression.

Consistent with the animal studies, human studies showed that the CD-associated frame-shift *NOD2* variant L1007fsinsC is associated with enhanced mucosal colonization by *Bacteroidetes* and *Firmicutes*[42] compared with the healthy controls. Another 2 human studies combined the 3 major CD risk alleles of *NOD2* (R702W, G908R, and L1007fsinsC) and confirmed that genotype and disease phenotype are associated with shifts in their intestinal microbial compositions.[46–48]

However, 2 recent studies[49,50] reported that only minimal differences were found in gut microbial composition between cohoused, littermate-controlled *NOD2*-deficient and wild-type mice, suggesting that the shifts in bacterial communities were not dependent on genotype but correlated with housing conditions. Although those findings might be partly explained by the restoration of disturbed microbiota because of animal cohousing, more studies are required to fully understand the role of *NOD2* in host-microbe interactions.

Similar to *NOD2/CARD15*, *NOD1/CARD4* also recognizes peptidoglycan found predominantly in gram-negative bacteria. In contrast to *NOD2*, CD susceptibility related to variants of the *NOD1* gene has been suggested but remains controversial.[51–53] One animal study showed that recognition of peptidoglycan from the microbiota by *NOD1*, not *NOD2*, primes systemic innate immunity by enhancing the cytotoxicity of bone-marrow derived neutrophils in response to systemic infection with the bacterial pathogens *Streptococcus pneumoniae* and *Staphylococcus aureus*.[54] However, the interplay between *NOD1* and gut microbiome has not been confirmed in human studies.

Autophagy

One of the major CD susceptibility genes, *ATG16L1* encodes a key component of the autophagy machinery to degrade damaged or obsolete organelles and proteins. Functional studies have shown that *ATG16L1* knockdown in intestinal epithelial cell lines impairs the clearance of *Salmonella typhimurium* infection.[55] In *ATG16L1* expression suppressed mice, studies have shown that microbial compositions were substantially shifted compared with the wild-type controls.[56] In humans, 2 case-control studies[47,48] on carriers with CD-associated *ATG16L1* risk allele T300A confirmed the significant association between host *ATG16L1* gene and the shift of gut microbiome profile.

Maintenance of Epithelial Barrier Integrity

Fucosyltransferase 2 (*FUT2*) is an enzyme that is responsible for the synthesis of the H antigen. The H antigen is an oligosaccharide moiety on the intestinal mucosa that acts as both an attachment site and carbon source for intestinal bacteria. The secretor status determines the expression of the ABH and Lewis histoblood group antigens in the intestinal mucosa. Nonsecretors, who are homozygous for the loss of function nonsense mutation of the *FUT2* gene, have shown increased susceptibility to CD.[57] Several human studies found that the host secretor status, encoded by *FUT2*, altered the intestinal microbiota composition.[7,58,59] Bifidobacterial diversity and abundance were significantly reduced in fecal samples from nonsecretors compared with those from the secretors.[59] The distinct clustering of the overall intestinal microbiota and significant differences in relative abundances of several dominant taxa, including *Clostridium* and *Blautia*, were observed between the nonsecretors and the secretors as well as between the *FUT2* genotypes.[58] In addition, the nonsecretors had lower species richness than the secretors.

Overall, the candidate gene approaches, in which the selected gene is deleted, suppressed, or overexpressed in an animal model or cell line, have shown the host genetic effect on modulating the structure and diversity of the gut microbiota. In addition, even with moderate sample size, emerging evidence from human studies has confirmed the interaction between host genetics and the gut microbiome, supporting the results from animal studies.

FUTURE PERSPECTIVES

CD is a complex disease resulting from both genetic predispositions and environmental factors, including the gut microbiota. Although distinctive membership and composition of the gut microbiota have been shown to play a significant role in CD pathogenesis, because of the sample size, human studies were limited to studying the effect of only 1 or 2 candidate genes on the gut microbiome of patients with CD and unaffected individuals based on the carriage status. Therefore, a large cohort is required to compare the bacterial distribution and abundance in the intestine of the patients with regard to disease status (CD vs no CD) and global genetic networks containing multiple CD risk loci. The gut microbiota profiles generated from this large cohort can be used to develop a predictive model combining both genetic and micro-biome signatures to assess the overall risk of CD among individuals. With a better understanding of the microbiome-host gene interplay associated with CD pathogen-esis, comprehensive diagnostic tools can be developed to identify individuals at risk for developing CD, as well as to develop novel personalized treatments.

REFERENCES

1. Abraham C, Cho JH. Inflammatory bowel disease. N Engl J Med 2009;361(21): 2066–78.
2. Scaldaferri F, Fiocchi C. Inflammatory bowel disease: progress and current con-cepts of etiopathogenesis. J Dig Dis 2007;8(4):171–8.
3. Yang H, Li Y, Wu W, et al. The incidence of inflammatory bowel disease in northern China: a prospective population-based study. PLoS One 2014;9(7):e101296.
4. Lakatos PL. Recent trends in the epidemiology of inflammatory bowel diseases: up or down? World J Gastroenterol 2006;12(38):6102–8.
5. Benchimol EI, Fortinsky KJ, Gozdyra P, et al. Epidemiology of pediatric inflam-matory bowel disease: a systematic review of international trends. Inflamm Bowel Dis 2011;17(1):423–39.
6. Loftus EV Jr. Clinical epidemiology of inflammatory bowel disease: incidence, prev-alence, and environmental influences. Gastroenterology 2004;126(6):1504–17.
7. Rausch P, Rehman A, Kunzel S, et al. Colonic mucosa-associated microbiota is influenced by an interaction of Crohn disease and FUT2 (secretor) genotype. Proc Natl Acad Sci U S A 2011;108(47):19030–5.
8. Jostins L, Ripke S, Weersma RK, et al. Host-microbe interactions have shaped the genetic architecture of inflammatory bowel disease. Nature 2012;491(7422): 119–24.
9. Vasseur F, Sendid B, Jouault T, et al. Variants of NOD1 and NOD2 genes display opposite associations with familial risk of Crohn's disease and anti–*Saccharo-myces cerevisiae* antibody levels. Inflamm Bowel Dis 2012;18(3):430–8.
10. Billmann-Born S, Till A, Arlt A, et al. Genome-wide expression profiling identifies an impairment of negative feedback signals in the Crohn's disease-associated NOD2 variant L1007fsinsC. J Immunol 2011;186(7):4027–38.
11. Cadwell K. Crohn's disease susceptibility gene interactions, a NOD to the newcomer ATG16L1. Gastroenterology 2010;139(5):1448–50.
12. Cooney R, Baker J, Brain O, et al. NOD2 stimulation induces autophagy in den-dritic cells influencing bacterial handling and antigen presentation. Nat Med 2010;16(1):90–7.
13. Homer CR, Richmond AL, Rebert NA, et al. ATG16L1 and NOD2 interact in an autophagy-dependent antibacterial pathway implicated in Crohn's disease pathogenesis. Gastroenterology 2010;139(5):1630–41, 1641.e1–2.
14. Hugot JP, Chamaillard M, Zouali H, et al. Association of NOD2 leucine-rich repeat variants with susceptibility to Crohn's disease. Nature 2001;411(6837): 599–603.

15. Kosovac K, Brenmoehl J, Holler E, et al. Association of the NOD2 genotype with bacterial translocation via altered cell-cell contacts in Crohn's disease patients. Inflamm Bowel Dis 2010;16(8):1311–21.

16. Ogura Y, Bonen DK, Inohara N, et al. A frameshift mutation in NOD2 associated with susceptibility to Crohn's disease. Nature 2001;411(6837):603–6.

17. Travassos LH, Carneiro LA, Ramjeet M, et al. Nod1 and Nod2 direct autophagy by recruiting ATG16L1 to the plasma membrane at the site of bacterial entry. Nat Immunol 2010;11(1):55–62.

18. Brest P, Lapaquette P, Mograbi B, et al. Risk predisposition for Crohn disease: a "menage a trois" combining IRGM allele, miRNA and xenophagy. Autophagy 2011;7(7):786–7.

19. Brest P, Lapaquette P, Souidi M, et al. A synonymous variant in IRGM alters a binding site for miR-196 and causes deregulation of IRGM-dependent xenophagy in Crohn's disease. Nat Genet 2011;43(3):242–5.

20. Parkes M, Barrett JC, Prescott NJ, et al. Sequence variants in the autophagy gene IRGM and multiple other replicating loci contribute to Crohn's disease susceptibility. Nat Genet 2007;39(7):830–2.

21. Hampe J, Franke A, Rosenstiel P, et al. A genome-wide association scan of non-synonymous SNPs identifies a susceptibility variant for Crohn disease in ATG16L1. Nat Genet 2007;39(2):207–11.

22. Gomez-Suaga P, Luzon-Toro B, Churamani D, et al. Leucine-rich repeat kinase 2 regulates autophagy through a calcium-dependent pathway involving NAADP. Hum Mol Genet 2012;21(3):511–25.

23. Friedrichs F, Stoll M. Role of discs large homolog 5. World J Gastroenterol 2006; 12(23):3651–6.

24. Tong M, McHardy I, Ruegger P, et al. Reprograming of gut microbiome energy metabolism by the FUT2 Crohn's disease risk polymorphism. ISME J 2014. [Epub ahead of print].

25. Somerville KW, Logan RF, Edmond M, et al. Smoking and Crohn's disease. BMJ 1984;289(6450):954–6.

26. Jakobsson HE, Jernberg C, Andersson AF, et al. Short-term antibiotic treatment has differing long-term impacts on the human throat and gut microbiome. PLoS One 2010;5(3):e9836.

27. Koren O, Spor A, Felin J, et al. Human oral, gut, and plaque microbiota in patients with atherosclerosis. Proc Natl Acad Sci U S A 2011;108(Suppl 1): 4592–8.

28. Savage DC. Microbial ecology of the gastrointestinal tract. Annu Rev Microbiol 1977;31:107–33.

29. Artis D. Epithelial-cell recognition of commensal bacteria and maintenance of immune homeostasis in the gut. Nat Rev Immunol 2008;8(6):411–20.

30. Gao Z, Tseng CH, Pei Z, et al. Molecular analysis of human forearm superficial skin bacterial biota. Proc Natl Acad Sci U S A 2007;104(8):2927–32.

31. Grice EA, Kong HH, Renaud G, et al. A diversity profile of the human skin microbiota. Genome Res 2008;18(7):1043–50.

32. Qin J, Li R, Raes J, et al. A human gut microbial gene catalogue established by metagenomic sequencing. Nature 2010;464(7285):59–65.

33. Turnbaugh PJ, Hamady M, Yatsunenko T, et al. A core gut microbiome in obese and lean twins. Nature 2009;457(7228):480–4.

34. Turnbaugh PJ, Ley RE, Hamady M, et al. The human microbiome project. Nature 2007;449(7164):804–10.

35. Turnbaugh PJ, Quince C, Faith JJ, et al. Organismal, genetic, and transcriptional variation in the deeply sequenced gut microbiomes of identical twins. Proc Natl Acad Sci U S A 2010;107(16):7503–8.

36. Hartman AL, Lough DM, Barupal DK, et al. Human gut microbiome adopts an alternative state following small bowel transplantation. Proc Natl Acad Sci U S A 2009;106(40):17187–92.

37. Manichanh C, Rigottier-Gois L, Bonnaud E, et al. Reduced diversity of faecal microbiota in Crohn's disease revealed by a metagenomic approach. Gut 2006;55(2):205–11.

38. Morgan XC, Tickle TL, Sokol H, et al. Dysfunction of the intestinal microbiome in inflammatory bowel disease and treatment. Genome Biol 2012;13(9):R79.

39. Gevers D, Kugathasan S, Denson LA, et al. The treatment-naive microbiome in new-onset Crohn's disease. Cell Host Microbe 2014;15(3):382–92.

40. Haberman Y, Tickle TL, Dexheimer PJ, et al. Pediatric Crohn disease patients exhibit specific ileal transcriptome and microbiome signature. J Clin Invest 2014;124(8):3617–33.

41. Petnicki-Ocwieja T, Hrncir T, Liu YJ, et al. Nod2 is required for the regulation of commensal microbiota in the intestine. Proc Natl Acad Sci U S A 2009;106(37): 15813–8.

42. Rehman A, Sina C, Gavrilova O, et al. Nod2 is essential for temporal development of intestinal microbial communities. Gut 2011;60(10):1354–62.

43. Couturier-Maillard A, Secher T, Rehman A, et al. NOD2-mediated dysbiosis predisposes mice to transmissible colitis and colorectal cancer. J Clin Invest 2013;123(2):700–11.

44. Smith P, Siddharth J, Pearson R, et al. Host genetics and environmental factors regulate ecological succession of the mouse colon tissue-associated microbiota. PLoS One 2012;7(1):e30273.

45. Voss E, Wehkamp J, Wehkamp K, et al. NOD2/CARD15 mediates induction of the antimicrobial peptide human beta-defensin-2. J Biol Chem 2006;281(4): 2005–11.

46. Frank DN, Robertson CE, Hamm CM, et al. Disease phenotype and genotype are associated with shifts in intestinal-associated microbiota in inflammatory bowel diseases. Inflamm Bowel Dis 2011;17(1):179–84.

47. Li E, Hamm CM, Gulati AS, et al. Inflammatory bowel diseases phenotype, *C. difficile* and NOD2 genotype are associated with shifts in human ileum associated microbial composition. PLoS One 2012;7(6):e26284.

48. Zhang T, DeSimone RA, Jiao X, et al. Host genes related to Paneth cells and xenobiotic metabolism are associated with shifts in human ileum-associated microbial composition. PLoS One 2012;7(6):e30044.

49. Shanahan MT, Carroll IM, Grossniklaus E, et al. Mouse Paneth cell antimicrobial function is independent of Nod2. Gut 2014;63(6):903–10.

50. Robertson SJ, Zhou JY, Geddes K, et al. Nod1 and Nod2 signaling does not alter the composition of intestinal bacterial communities at homeostasis. Gut Microbes 2013;4(3):222–31.

51. McGovern DP, Hysi P, Ahmad T, et al. Association between a complex insertion/deletion polymorphism in NOD1 (CARD4) and susceptibility to inflammatory bowel disease. Hum Mol Genet 2005;14(10):1245–50.

52. Van Limbergen J, Russell RK, Nimmo ER, et al. Contribution of the NOD1/CARD4 insertion/deletion polymorphism +32656 to inflammatory bowel disease in Northern Europe. Inflamm Bowel Dis 2007;13(7):882–9.

53. Zouali H, Lesage S, Merlin F, et al. CARD4/NOD1 is not involved in inflammatory bowel disease. Gut 2003;52(1):71–4.
54. Clarke TB, Davis KM, Lysenko ES, et al. Recognition of peptidoglycan from the microbiota by Nod1 enhances systemic innate immunity. Nat Med 2010;16(2): 228–31.
55. Rioux JD, Xavier RJ, Taylor KD, et al. Genome-wide association study identifies new susceptibility loci for Crohn disease and implicates autophagy in disease pathogenesis. Nat Genet 2007;39(5):596–604.
56. Simmons A. Crohn's disease: genes, viruses and microbes. Nature 2010; 466(7307):699–700.
57. McGovern DP, Jones MR, Taylor KD, et al. Fucosyltransferase 2 (FUT2) non-secretor status is associated with Crohn's disease. Hum Mol Genet 2010; 19(17):3468–76.
58. Wacklin P, Tuimala J, Nikkila J, et al. Faecal microbiota composition in adults is associated with the FUT2 gene determining the secretor status. PLoS One 2014; 9(4):e94863.
59. Wacklin P, Makivuokko H, Alakulppi N, et al. Secretor genotype (FUT2 gene) is strongly associated with the composition of *Bifidobacteria* in the human intestine. PLoS One 2011;6(5):e20113.

The Impact of Proton Pump Inhibitors on the Human Gastrointestinal Microbiome

 CrossMark

Daniel E. Freedberg, MD, MS[a],[*], Benjamin Lebwohl, MD, MS[a],[b], Julian A. Abrams, MD, MS[a]

KEYWORDS

- Proton pump inhibitors • Gastric acid suppression • Hypergastrinemia
- Human microbiome • Barrett's esophagus • *Helicobacter pylori*
- Small bowel bacterial overgrowth • *Clostridium difficile* infection

KEY POINTS

- Proton pump inhibitors (PPIs) have the potential to affect human health via interactions with the gastrointestinal microbiome.
- PPIs reduce esophageal gram-negative bacteria and may decrease risk for distal esophageal neoplasia.
- Given for *Helicobacter pylori* eradication, PPIs can prevent gastric cancer but may cause gastric dysbiosis after *H pylori* has been eradicated.
- PPIs may cause small intestinal bacterial overgrowth and are associated with the diagnosis of celiac disease.
- PPIs are associated with *Clostridium difficile* infection (CDI), although the mechanism linking PPIs and CDI is uncertain.

INTRODUCTION

For centuries, it has been known that dietary factors influence gastrointestinal bacteria; Dorlencourt and Lavaudon[1] hypothesized that pH differences between breast milk and cow's milk explained the higher proportions of *Lactobacillus* observed in the

Funding: D.E. Freedberg was supported in part by National Institutes of Health training grants (T32 DK083256 and UL1 RR024156); B. Lebwohl was supported in part by The National Center for Advancing Translational Sciences, NIH (UL1 TR000040) and the American Gastroenterological Association Research Scholar Award; J.A. Abrams was supported in part by Columbia University's Irving Scholar Award and an NIH grant (U54 CA 163004).
Financial Disclosures: The authors have nothing to disclose.
[a] Division of Digestive and Liver Diseases, Columbia University Medical Center, 630 West 168th Street, New York, NY 10032, USA; [b] Celiac Disease Center at Columbia University, 180 Fort Washington Avenue, New York, NY 10032, USA
* Corresponding author. Division of Digestive and Liver Diseases, Columbia University Medical Center, 630 West 168th Street, PH Building, Floor 7, New York, NY 10032.
E-mail address: def2004@cumc.columbia.edu

stools of breastfed children. The role of gastric acidity in the human gastrointestinal microbiome is now intertwined with the development and increasing use of proton pump inhibitors (PPIs). Other medications can alter the pH of the human gastrointestinal lumen. However, PPIs are the most potent, the most common, and have received the most attention. This article focuses on PPIs and covers the physiology of gastric acid production and suppression, and the evidence and clinical consequences of acid-related changes in the normal microbiome.

PROTON PUMP INHIBITORS AND GASTROINTESTINAL ACIDITY
Normal Gastrointestinal Acidity

Acidity within the human gastrointestinal tract varies by anatomic location and is part of essential physiologic processes, including digestion and nutrient absorption.[2] In the stomach, lumenal pH can approach 1.0; gastric acid plays a role in breakdown of food particles and the pH-dependent separation of intrinsic factor from R-protein.[3] Outside the stomach, lumenal pH is often discussed in the context of optimizing drug delivery. In general, pH tends to increase gradually from 6.5 in the small bowel to a high of 7.5, decrease in the cecum (to as low as 5.5), and again increase gradually in the left colon to a high of 6.5 to 7.0.[4] The invariant pattern of gastrointestinal pH seen between individuals suggests that pH plays crucial physiologic roles throughout the gastrointestinal tract. Local pH partially determines the absorption of biotin and folate in the small bowel,[5,6] vitamin B_{12} in the distal ileum,[7] and calcium and other electrolytes in the colon.[8] Thus, in addition to the influence that pH exerts on the microbiome, gastrointestinal acidity is important and tightly regulated.

Physiology of Gastric Acid Production

Food, stress, and other central and hormonal mechanisms stimulate gastric acid secretion acting via autonomic and paracrine signals. The primary signals are gastrin from pyloric and duodenal G cells, acetylcholine from postganglionic neurons in the gastric submucosa, and histamine from enterochromaffinlike cells; the common target of these signals and the acid-producing cells of the stomach is the parietal cell.[9] In response to stimuli, transmembrane H^+/K^+-ATPase pumps are translocated from tubulovesicles into parietal cell canaliculi, increasing their concentration on the cell surface by 10-fold. These powerful pumps then acidify the stomach by using ATP for energy to drive protons or hydronium ions against enormous concentration gradients.[10]

Proton Pump Inhibitors

PPIs were independently synthesized by 2 companies from 2-pyridylthioacetamide by screening modified compounds (**Fig. 1**); the first PPIs were omeprazole (1988) and lansoprazole (1991).[11] There were initial safety concerns surrounding omeprazole, which

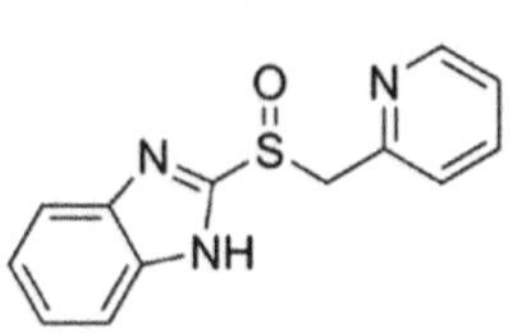

Fig. 1. Common structure of PPIs. All PPIs share a common backbone, with a pyridine linked to a benzimidazole.

was linked to increased risk for gastric carcinoids.[12] Subsequent studies suggested that PPIs did not confer increased risk for malignancy and more PPIs were developed, including enantiomers (esomeprazole and dexlansoprazole) of the original PPIs.[13] There are currently 7 PPIs available in the United States by prescription, 2 PPIs (omeprazole and lansoprazole) that are available over the counter, and 3 PPIs (omeprazole, lansoprazole, and pantoprazole) that are available as generics. Because PPIs are metabolized through the hepatic cytochrome P450 system, drug levels can vary between formulations for individuals with certain pharmacogenetic characteristics.[14] However, there is little evidence that the various PPI formulations differ significantly in clinical efficacy or in side effects.[15]

All PPIs are prodrugs that are concentrated in a pH-dependent manner in the canaliculi of parietal cells. PPIs are concentrated within acidic parietal cell canaliculi, protonated, and covalently bound to cysteine residues of parietal cell H^+/K^+-ATPase antiporter pumps.[16] Because stimulation at the prospect of food causes H^+/K^+-ATPases to be translocated into parietal cell canaliculi, PPIs are most effective if taken before meals when the maximal number of H^+/K^+-ATPases are available as targets. Once bound by PPIs, parietal cell H^+/K^+-ATPases are irreversibly fixed into an inactive configuration, which lasts approximately 24 hours until more H^+/K^+-ATPases can be inserted from resting intracellular vesicles into the apical membrane of the parietal cell. The key to the high efficacy of PPIs is that they inhibit the end pathway of gastric acid production and thus, unlike other acid-suppressive medications, cannot be overwhelmed by normal physiologic compensatory mechanisms.

In the stomach, PPIs induce profound hypochlorhydria. Serum concentration peaks after 2 to 5 hours; after 3 to 4 hours, a single oral PPI dose increases gastric pH in most patients from 2.0 to more than 6.0; a 10,000-fold change.[17] The pH-increasing effect of PPIs persists in the proximal duodenum, but is attenuated by the distal duodenum. In a study of healthy volunteers who underwent continuous pH monitoring, median pH in the distal duodenum was 5.85 after 1 week of PPIs compared with 5.95 after 1 week of placebo.[18] Using wireless capsule pH measurement, there is similar overall small bowel pH between users and nonusers of high-dose PPIs.[19] The best available evidence thus suggests that, by the proximal jejunum, the direct pH effect of PPIs has been fully attenuated and is no longer significant.

PPIs have established clinical efficacy for many health conditions, including peptic ulcer disease, gastroesophageal reflux, eosinophilic esophagitis, and acid hypersecretory conditions (eg, Zollinger-Ellison syndrome). Because they are effective and are thought to be benign, PPIs have gained widespread use. They are perennially among the top 3 drug classes by sales in the world; one PPI, esomeprazole, was the fourth most prescribed drug by sales in the United States in 2012 and the top drug by sales through the first 6 months of 2013.[20] When used for appropriate indications, PPIs have great benefits. However, they are often prescribed in situations in which they have no potential clinical benefit.[21] More than half of all inpatients who receive PPIs do not have an appropriate indication for the drugs and, among these patients, more than one-third are discharged on PPIs.[22] Among outpatients, 80% of PPI prescriptions are repeats and 40% to 50% are for nonspecific abdominal pain.[23]

Non–pH-dependent Effects of Proton Pump Inhibitors

The influence of PPIs on the gastrointestinal microbiome is presumed to depend on their capacity to increase gastric pH. However, PPIs also have the potential to influence the microbiome through pH-independent mechanisms. First, PPIs induce hormonal changes, including hypergastrinemia and hyperparathyroidism, which have the potential to alter the gastrointestinal bacterial milieu.[24] Second, PPIs can alter lumenal contents to interfere with nutrient absorption and change the amount or location of bacterial food substrates. Case reports and cross-sectional studies document increased hypomagnesemia among patients on long-term PPIs, suggesting the possibility that PPIs interfere with small bowel magnesium transport.[25,26] In addition, PPIs have been shown to bind nongastric H^+/K^+-ATPases, both on human cells and on commensal bacteria and fungi.[27] The P-type family of ATPases, which includes H^+/K^+-ATPases, is present on fungi, *Helicobacter pylori*,[28] and *Streptococcus pneumoniae*,[29] but little is known about the effect of PPIs on specific bacteria aside from *H pylori*.

EFFECTS OF PROTON PUMP INHIBITORS ON THE MICROBIOME
Esophagus

PPIs are first-line treatment of acid-related esophageal disorders, including gastroesophageal reflux disease (GERD), erosive esophagitis, Barrett's esophagus (BE), suspected eosinophilic esophagitis, and nonerosive reflux disease.[30–32] Esophageal disorders are the most common reason for prescribing a PPI. Since the 1970s, there has been a 5-fold to 10-fold increase in BE and esophageal adenocarcinoma (EAC), with a parallel increase in GERD.[33,34] In a large pharmacy database, more than 60% of patients on long-term PPIs reported heartburn and 68% carried diagnoses of GERD, dyspepsia, or both.[35] However, diagnostic testing was rare; only 27% of these patients underwent upper endoscopy and only 3% had testing for *H pylori*.

The esophageal microbiome is altered in esophagitis and BE compared with normal controls.[36] A study of distal esophageal specimens from 34 subjects who had esophagitis, BE, or an endoscopically normal esophagus found that the microbiome could be separated into 2 types: a pattern dominated by *Streptococcus* that associated with a normal esophagus, and a pattern dominated by gram-negative anaerobes or microaerophilic bacteria that associated with esophagitis or Barrett's. These gram-negative bacteria may increase esophageal inflammation by activating Toll-like receptor 4 and the nuclear factor kappa B (NF-κB) pathway through surface lipopolysaccharides.[37] An alternative is that these bacteria may increase distal esophageal acid exposure by decreasing lower esophageal sphincter tone or by delaying gastric emptying.[38,39]

PPIs are thought to protect against progression of BE to EAC by decreasing distal esophageal mucosal acid exposure. PPIs simultaneously alter the distal esophageal microbiome in ways that may affect inflammation and carcinogenesis. The mucosal-associated microbiota of the distal esophagus, which is altered in patients with esophagitis or BE,[36,40] is further modified by PPIs. A study of 34 patients with Barrett's, esophagitis, or a normal distal esophagus used 16S ribosomal RNA (rRNA) gene sequencing to assess the microbiome from distal esophageal biopsies and gastric aspirates, comparing results before versus after PPIs.[41] Before PPIs were administered, there were no major differences in distal esophageal mucosal bacteria between patients with esophagitis/BE and controls. After PPIs were administered, there were significant increases in distal esophageal Lachnospiraceae, Comamonadaceae, and unclassified clostridial families. The family Methylobacteriaceae, which were increased in gastric aspirates among patients with BE/esophagitis before PPIs, were highly depleted in these patients after PPI therapy. This bacterial family has also been associated with inflamed tissue in patients with inflammatory bowel disease and found in patients with irritable bowel syndrome, suggesting that these bacteria can only thrive on altered mucosa.[42]

Although *Helicobacter* is not a dominant organism in the esophagus, *H pylori* exerts control over the distal esophageal microbiome. There is a strong inverse correlation between *H pylori* infection (especially *cag*A-positive *H pylori*) and BE or EAC.[43,44] A recent study by Fischbach and colleagues[45] investigated the role of acid suppression in the *H pylori*–Barrett relationship. The odds ratio for the association between *H pylori* and BE was 0.56 among those who used PPIs compared with 0.90 among those who did not, implying that PPIs augment the protective effects of *H pylori* for BE. These results are surprising because PPIs have powerful anti–*H pylori* activity and *H pylori* seems to be protective for esophageal neoplasia. The most likely explanation is that the direct protective effects of PPIs in Barrett's (via decreased distal esophageal acid exposure) outweigh indirect and less potent anti–*H pylori* effects. Future studies should further elaborate the influence of PPIs in the *H pylori*–Barrett relationship and determine the precise mechanisms by which PPIs alter the distal esophageal microbiome.

Stomach

PPIs are a mainstay of *H pylori* eradication therapy and have direct bacteriostatic activity against *H pylori*[46] as well as indirect *Helicobacter* activity via increases in gastric pH. Because *H pylori* and an acidic environment are necessary for the formation of most gastric and duodenal ulcers, PPIs effectively prevent peptic ulcer disease and greatly speed the healing of ulcers that have already formed.[47] PPIs are often used in nonulcer dyspepsia and other functional gastric conditions, although their utility under these circumstances is less clear.

The acidity of the stomach distinguishes the gastric niche from the rest of the human gastrointestinal tract and determines the composition of the gastric flora. *H pylori* is the dominant microorganism of the stomach, accounting for at least 70% of the gastric microbiome by 16S rRNA sequencing in positive individuals.[48] Gastric acidity both allows *H pylori* to thrive and is influenced by the presence of *H pylori*. Acid suppression with PPIs decreases *H pylori* abundance and, in antrum-predominant infection, shifts the location of *H pylori* to the corpus; meanwhile, corpus-predominant *H pylori* infection can cause atrophic gastritis and achlorhydria.[49]

PPIs cause gastric bacterial overgrowth, and PPI-induced gastric bacterial overgrowth is related to *H pylori* infection. Individuals infected with *H pylori* have greater pH changes with PPIs than do uninfected individuals and they are consequently more susceptible to overgrowth.[50] When *H pylori* is absent, dominant gastric bacteria include oral flora such as *Streptococcus* (primarily in the mitis group)[51] and common commensals such as *Lactobacillus* and *Clostridium* spp, which occur elsewhere in the gastrointestinal tract.[52,53] When gastric pH is increased to more than 4.0 by PPIs, *Lactobacillus* spp, *Streptococcus* spp, and other gastric bacteria proliferate and can cause nausea, bloating, and altered concentrations of upper gastrointestinal anaerobes, which in turn affects conjugation of bile acids and can lead to diarrhea.[54,55]

In susceptible individuals, chronic *H pylori* infection leads to multifocal atrophic gastritis, gastric epithelial dysplasia, and gastric cancer.[56] This stepwise inflammatory process, termed the Correa cascade, has been shown in animal models and corroborated by human studies; in 1994, *H pylori* was recognized as a class I (definite) carcinogen by the World Health Organization.[57] Because of improved hygiene and increased use of antibiotics, *H pylori* infection is declining in the developed world. However, in areas at high risk for gastric cancer, PPIs have been successfully used with antibiotics to eradicate *H pylori* for the chemoprevention of gastric cancer. Two large, randomized, and placebo-controlled trials have been conducted in areas in China with very high baseline rates of gastric cancer. The first study, conducted among 1630 participants with *H pylori* infection in the Fujian province showed that antibiotics and PPIs decreased incident gastric cancer among those without precursor lesions after

7.5 years of follow-up.[58] A second, larger trial in the Shandong province showed a significant reduction in incident gastric cancer among all participants, comparing PPIs and amoxicillin versus placebo after 15 years of follow-up.[59] Because of these and similar data, short courses of PPIs are recommended as part of a chemopreventive strategy in high-risk individuals with *H pylori* infection in guidelines from the United States, Europe, and Asia.[47,60,61]

In *H pylori*–negative individuals, the effect of chronic PPI use on gastric dysplasia is less clear, and recent data suggest that *H pylori* is not the only gastric microorganism that contributes to dysplasia and gastric cancer. *H pylori* does not thrive in the high-pH environment associated with gastric cancer. In patients with gastric cancer, *H pylori* decreases in abundance and there is a shift toward streptococci genera that are not often found in normal individuals.[62] Recent data from mouse models have contributed to understanding of the role of the non–*H pylori* gastric microbiome in the pathogenesis of gastric cancer, although the high gastric pH of mice (baseline 3.0–4.0) may limit the ability to generalize murine microbiome findings to humans.[63] A well-established mouse model of gastric cancer is the transgenic INS-GAS mouse, which overexpresses gastrin and almost invariably develops gastric cancer.[64] When raised in a germ-free environment, *H pylori*–monoinfected INS-GAS mice had delayed progression of gastric dysplasia compared with mice with a complex gastric microbiome.[65] Introduction of complex microbiota or of defined species (altered Schaedler flora) into the stomachs of INS-GAS mice was sufficient to accelerate dysplasia.[66] This finding raises the possibility that PPIs, if continued after *H pylori* eradication, could promote gastric cancer pathogenesis by causing non–*H pylori* gastric dysbiosis that perpetuates the Correa cascade.

The preponderance of data does not support the idea that PPIs accelerate cancer in the stomach in humans through the microbiome or other mechanisms. Early animal studies of omeprazole showed increased rates of enterochromaffin cell carcinoids, but subsequent lifelong studies of rats failed to confirm this finding.[12] Further animal studies did not indicate risk,[13] and long-term prospective cohort data in humans have not shown an association between PPIs and gastric carcinoids or gastric adenocarcinoma.[67]

Small Bowel

The profound effect of PPIs on pH is limited to the stomach and proximal duodenum, with little to no effect on the pH of most of the small bowel.[18] Nevertheless, gastric acid suppression by PPIs exerts a downstream effect on small intestinal bacterial composition. The increase in the quantity and diversity of the gastric microbiome in PPI users is paralleled by an increase in the quantity of bacteria in the proximal small bowel. A study of 450 consecutive patients undergoing glucose hydrogen breath test for suspected small intestinal bacterial overgrowth (SIBO) found that 50% of PPI users tested positively, compared with 6% of nonusers.[68] Using duodenal aspirates and a diagnostic criterion of 10^3 colonic-type organisms per milliliter of fluid, a study of more than 300 patients found that 36% of PPI users had SIBO compared with 22% of nonusers.[69] The most common organisms in patients with SIBO were *Escherichia coli* (37%), *Enterococcus* spp (32%), and *Klebsiella pneumoniae* (24%). In addition, a recent meta-analysis found a nearly 3-fold increase in the risk of SIBO among adult users of PPIs compared with nonusers (odds ratio [OR], 2.28; 95% confidence interval [CI], 1.24–4.21).[70] The association was particularly strong when the end point of SIBO was classified solely on the gold standard of duodenal or jejunal aspirates (OR, 7.59). Although individuals with SIBO are often asymptomatic, clinical sequelae can include gas and bloating sensations caused by increased intraluminal carbohydrate fermentation, iron and vitamin B_{12} deficiency caused by competitive microbial uptake, and fat malabsorption as a consequence of bacterial deconjugation of bile acids.[71,72]

PPIs are often prescribed to provide gastric protection in patients who are coingesting nonsteroidal antiinflammatory drugs (NSAIDs), but the combined use of these agents may exert a paradoxic cytotoxic effect on the small bowel. In a study of rats administered omeprazole or lansoprazole for 9 days plus celecoxib or naproxen for the final 4 days, PPI use was associated with reductions in jejunal Actinobacteria and Bifidobacteria, and exacerbated intestinal damage.[73] This injury seemed to be mediated by dysbiosis, because injury was ameliorated when PPI-treated rats were repleted with a Bifidobacteria-enriched microbiota. Also, when germ-free mice were given jejunal bacteria from PPI-treated rats, the germ-free mice had more severe NSAID-related injuries than the germ-free mice given bacteria from control rats. Although this effect has not been shown in humans, these results suggest that PPIs, when coadministered with NSAIDs, may potentiate cytotoxicity in the small bowel via a microbiome-mediated effect.

The increase of PPI use in recent decades has coincided temporally with an increased incidence of celiac disease, an immune-mediated enteropathy characterized by intraepithelial lymphocytosis and villous atrophy in response to the ingestion of gluten. Children with celiac disease seem to have distinct duodenal microbial characteristics, including reduced *Lactobacillus* and *Bifidobacterium* and increased *Bacteroides* and *E coli*.[74] A population-based case-control study found that a prescription of a PPI was far more likely in patients before being diagnosed with celiac disease compared with age-matched and sex-matched controls (OR, 4.79; 95% CI, 4.17–5.51). Given the possibility that PPIs may have been prescribed in response to symptoms of undiagnosed celiac disease, a sensitivity analysis excluding all PPI prescriptions in the 1 year immediately preceding this diagnosis found that the effect, although diminished, remained significant (OR, 2.28; 95% CI, 1.67–3.10).[75] Although these results do not prove causality, the potentially mediating effect of the microbiome on the PPI–celiac disease relationship warrants further investigation.

A second link between PPI use and the increased risk of celiac disease may relate to the effect of PPIs on *H pylori*. In a large cross-sectional study of simultaneously submitted gastric and duodenal biopsy specimens to a national commercial pathology laboratory, there was a strong inverse association between *H pylori* and celiac disease; this remained significant after adjusting for age, gender, and socioeconomic status (OR, 0.48; 95% CI, 0.40–0.58).[76] This apparently protective effect of *H pylori* may be caused by the local recruitment of regulatory T lymphocytes, damping the immune response to potentially antigenic dietary exposures.[77] Because PPIs exert a bacteriostatic effect on *H pylori*, the potentially protective effect of this bacterium on celiac disease risk may be diminished by PPIs; in support of this hypothesis, the increase in diagnosis of celiac disease correlates with decreased rates of *Helicobacter* infection in Western societies.

Colon

The large intestine contains most of the human gastrointestinal microbiome in part because the colonic pH of 5.5 to 7.0 permits the growth of many microbial species.[78] Elegant interspecies experiments show that, when a mammalian microbiome is transplanted into a germ-free zebrafish, the microbial structure quickly changes to resemble a conventional zebrafish microbiome.[79] This suggests that basic host characteristics (pH, temperature, and motility) are important determinants of overall microbiome structure. PPIs do not directly alter the pH of the colon, but they may have clinically important effects on the distal gut, and interest has focused on the relationship between PPIs and *Clostridium difficile* infection (CDI).

C difficile infection is a highly morbid form of infectious colitis that has been associated with exposure to PPIs in more than 30 observational studies.[80,81] During a period of declining use of antibiotics, the increase in CDI correlates with increased use of PPIs (**Fig. 2**).[82] An association between PPIs and CDI has been found among outpatients,[83] inpatients,[84] and patients in intensive care units.[85] Multiple meta-analyses and population-based data support these findings.[80,81] A program of active surveillance undertaken by the Centers for Disease Control and Prevention that covers more than 11 million people found that PPI exposure was 5% higher among those with CDI who did not report exposure to antibiotics, compared with those with CDI who did report exposure to antibiotics.[86]

The mechanism linking PPIs and CDI is uncertain, but is thought to be via the microbiome. *C difficile* spores are acid resistant, and acid suppression has little impact on their survival.[87,88] Antibiotic use causes CDI by depleting commensal bacteria that normally block *C difficile* proliferation and by reducing the diversity of the colonic microbiome.[89,90] PPIs cause small intestinal bacterial overgrowth with predominantly colonic species; it follows that, with overgrowth in the proximal gut, an altered bacterial load is delivered to the colon that may predispose to CDI. Distal gut bacteria interact with colonic epithelial cells and patients using PPIs have been shown to have increased colonic intraepithelial leukocytes[91] and fecal calprotectin levels,[92] suggesting colonic mucosal inflammation. PPIs may also directly bind colonic epithelial H^+/K^+-ATPases, or act on the colonic mucosa through NF-κB or other systemic immune pathways.[93] Further evidence supporting the hypothesis that the microbiome mediates the PPI-CDI relationship can be found in studies examining PPIs as a risk factor for recurrent CDI. Unlike studies of incident CDI, the relationship between PPIs and recurrent CDI is not clear.[94,95] It is biologically plausible that PPIs cause incident CDI by altering the colonic microbiome and that this effect is blunted after the microbiome has already been perturbed by CDI.

Few studies have investigated the changes within the fecal microbiome that precede CDI. In a prospective cohort study of 599 patients during a *C difficile* outbreak,

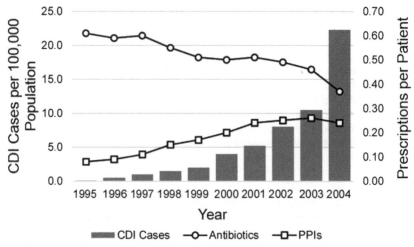

Fig. 2. Corresponding increases in the incidence of CDI and rate of PPI use, during a time of decreasing antibiotic use. (*Adapted from* Dial S, Delaney JA, Barkun AN, et al. Use of gastric acid-suppressive agents and the risk of community-acquired *Clostridium difficile*-associated disease. JAMA 2005;294(23):2989–95.)

decreased Bacteroidetes at the time of admission was associated with subsequent development of CDI.[96] When 16S rRNA sequencing was used to compare the fecal microbiomes from 25 patients who developed CDI with 25 randomly selected controls who did not, the patients who developed CDI had significant depletions in Clostridiales Incertae Sedis XI, a family that belongs to the same order as *C difficile*.[97] In humans, the combination of antibiotics and PPIs produced a pattern of reduced fecal bacterial diversity and reduced Bacteroidetes abundance, although the effect of PPIs alone in humans is unknown.[98]

Under controlled conditions, PPIs have effects on the fecal microbiome of animals. In dogs, administration of high-dose PPIs increased *Lactobacillus* and, in male dogs, reduced commensal fecal bacterial types including Bacteroidetes.[99] Another study used quantitative real-time polymerase chain reaction to assess the effect of achlorhydria on the fecal microbiome in Wistar rats treated with high-dose PPIs and humans with chronic atrophic gastritis.[100] There were significant increases in the levels of *Lactobacillus* in acid-suppressed rats and achlorhydric humans compared with controls, without comparable increases in Bacteroidetes. These fecal microbiome changes resemble some of the alterations seen after administration of antibiotics, raising the possibility that PPIs may act like antibiotics to decrease microbiome diversity or otherwise alter normal microbiome structure and decrease normal colonization resistance to *C difficile*.[90]

SUMMARY

PPIs irreversibly bind and inactivate gastric H^+/K^+-ATPases to induce profound gastric achlorhydria. PPIs are a highly effective treatment of acid-related disorders but are widely overused. PPIs alter the microbiome throughout the human gastrointestinal tract with important potential consequences for human health (**Fig. 3**). The ability of PPIs to heal erosive esophagitis and slow progression of BE may be partly mediated

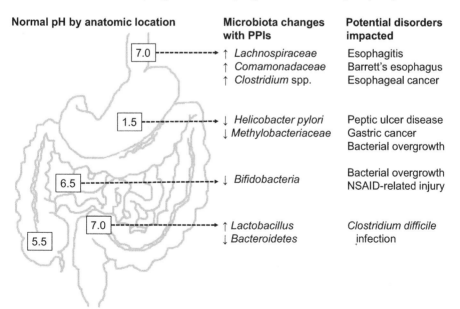

Fig. 3. Bacteria that may be affected by PPIs are shown by anatomic area; small arrows indicate directionality of changes with PPIs.

by PPI-related decreases in gram-negative bacteria. In the stomach, PPIs have a chemopreventive effect when used for eradication of *H pylori*, but contribute to gastric carcinogenesis in animals by causing dysbiosis if given after *H pylori* is eradicated. In the small bowel, PPIs may cause diarrhea through bacterial overgrowth and may be a risk factor for celiac disease. In addition, epidemiologic studies show that PPIs are associated with *C difficile* infection, although the mechanism linking PPIs and incident *C difficile* remains unclear. Further research is needed to determine the effect of PPIs on the gastrointestinal microbiome and on human health.

REFERENCES

1. Dorlencourt H, Lavaudon R. Les pH des selles des nourrissons sains et malades. Nourrisson 1931;19:147–53.
2. Evans DF, Pye G, Bramley R, et al. Measurement of gastrointestinal pH profiles in normal ambulant human subjects. Gut 1988;29(8):1035–41.
3. Berk L, Castle WB, Welch AD, et al. Observations on the etiologic relationship of achylia gastrica to pernicious anemia; activity of vitamin B12 as food, extrinsic factor. N Engl J Med 1948;239(24):911–3.
4. Fallingborg J. Intraluminal pH of the human gastrointestinal tract. Dan Med Bull 1999;46(3):183–96.
5. Said HM, Redha R, Nylander W. Biotin transport in the human intestine: site of maximum transport and effect of pH. Gastroenterology 1988;95(5):1312–7.
6. Strum WB. Enzymatic reduction and methylation of folate following pH-dependent, carrier-mediated transport in rat jejunum. Biochim Biophys Acta 1979;554(1): 249–57.
7. Lam JR, Schneider JL, Zhao W, et al. Proton pump inhibitor and histamine 2 receptor antagonist use and vitamin B12 deficiency. JAMA 2013;310(22):2435–42.
8. Carmel R, Rosenberg AH, Lau KS, et al. Vitamin B12 uptake by human small bowel homogenate and its enhancement by intrinsic factor. Gastroenterology 1969;56(3):548–55.
9. Feldman M, Friedman LS, Sleisenger MH. Sleisenger & Fordtran's gastrointestinal and liver disease: pathophysiology, diagnosis, management. 7th edition. Philadelphia: Saunders; 2002.
10. Munson K, Lambrecht N, Shin JM, et al. Analysis of the membrane domain of the gastric H(+)/K(+)-ATPase. J Exp Biol 2000;203(Pt 1):161–70.
11. Chiba T, Malfertheiner P, Satoh H. Proton pump inhibitors: a balanced view. Basel (Switzerland): Karger AG; 2013.
12. Larsson H, Carlsson E, Mattsson H, et al. Plasma gastrin and gastric enterochromaffinlike cell activation and proliferation. Studies with omeprazole and ranitidine in intact and antrectomized rats. Gastroenterology 1986;90(2):391–9.
13. Olbe L, Carlsson E, Lindberg P. A proton-pump inhibitor expedition: the case histories of omeprazole and esomeprazole. Nat Rev Drug Discov 2003;2(2): 132–9.
14. Sim SC, Risinger C, Dahl ML, et al. A common novel CYP2C19 gene variant causes ultrarapid drug metabolism relevant for the drug response to proton pump inhibitors and antidepressants. Clin Pharmacol Ther 2006;79(1):103–13.
15. Kahrilas PJ, Shaheen NJ, Vaezi MF, et al. American Gastroenterological Association Medical Position Statement on the management of gastroesophageal reflux disease. Gastroenterology 2008;135(4):1383–91, 1391.e1–5.
16. Shin JM, Munson K, Vagin O, et al. The gastric HK-ATPase: structure, function, and inhibition. Pflugers Arch 2009;457(3):609–22.

17. Laine L, Shah A, Bemanian S. Intragastric pH with oral vs intravenous bolus plus infusion proton-pump inhibitor therapy in patients with bleeding ulcers. Gastroenterology 2008;134(7):1836–41.

18. Gan KH, Geus WP, Lamers CB, et al. Effect of omeprazole 40 mg once daily on intraduodenal and intragastric pH in *H. pylori*-negative healthy subjects. Dig Dis Sci 1997;42(11):2304–9.

19. Michalek W, Semler JR, Kuo B. Impact of acid suppression on upper gastrointestinal pH and motility. Dig Dis Sci 2011;56(6):1735–42.

20. IMS Health. Top-Line Market Data. Available at: http://www.imshealth.com/portal/site/ims/menuitem.5ad1c081663fdf9b41d84b903208c22a/?vgnextoid=fbc65890d33ee210VgnVCM10000071812ca2RCRD. Accessed March 23, 2014.

21. Heidelbaugh JJ, Goldberg KL, Inadomi JM. Overutilization of proton pump inhibitors: a review of cost-effectiveness and risk [corrected]. Am J Gastroenterol 2009;104(Suppl 2):S27–32.

22. Zink DA, Pohlman M, Barnes M, et al. Long-term use of acid suppression started inappropriately during hospitalization. Aliment Pharmacol Ther 2005;21(10):1203–9.

23. Bashford JN, Norwood J, Chapman SR. Why are patients prescribed proton pump inhibitors? Retrospective analysis of link between morbidity and prescribing in the General Practice Research Database. BMJ 1998;317(7156):452–6.

24. Yang YX, Metz DC. Safety of proton pump inhibitor exposure. Gastroenterology 2010;139(4):1115–27.

25. Epstein M, McGrath S, Law F. Proton-pump inhibitors and hypomagnesemic hypoparathyroidism. N Engl J Med 2006;355(17):1834–6.

26. Markovits N, Loebstein R, Halkin H, et al. The association of proton pump inhibitors and hypomagnesemia in the community setting. J Clin Pharmacol 2014;54:889–95.

27. Vesper BJ, Jawdi A, Altman KW, et al. The effect of proton pump inhibitors on the human microbiota. Curr Drug Metab 2009;10(1):84–9.

28. Melchers K, Herrmann L, Mauch F, et al. Properties and function of the P type ion pumps cloned from *Helicobacter pylori*. Acta Physiol Scand Suppl 1998;643:123–35.

29. Hoskins J, Alborn WE Jr, Arnold J, et al. Genome of the bacterium *Streptococcus pneumoniae* strain R6. J Bacteriol 2001;183(19):5709–17.

30. Katz PO, Gerson LB, Vela MF. Guidelines for the diagnosis and management of gastroesophageal reflux disease. Am J Gastroenterol 2013;108(3):308–28 [quiz: 329].

31. Kahrilas PJ, Shaheen NJ, Vaezi MF, American Gastroenterological Association Institute, Clinical Practice and Quality Management Committee. American Gastroenterological Association Institute technical review on the management of gastroesophageal reflux disease. Gastroenterology 2008;135(4):1392–413, 1413.e1–5.

32. Dellon ES, Gonsalves N, Hirano I, et al. ACG clinical guideline: evidenced based approach to the diagnosis and management of esophageal eosinophilia and eosinophilic esophagitis (EoE). Am J Gastroenterol 2013;108(5):679–92 [quiz: 693].

33. El-Serag HB. Time trends of gastroesophageal reflux disease: a systematic review. Clin Gastroenterol Hepatol 2007;5(1):17–26.

34. Pohl H, Welch HG. The role of overdiagnosis and reclassification in the marked increase of esophageal adenocarcinoma incidence. J Natl Cancer Inst 2005;97(2):142–6.

35. Jacobson BC, Ferris TG, Shea TL, et al. Who is using chronic acid suppression therapy and why? Am J Gastroenterol 2003;98(1):51–8.

36. Yang L, Lu X, Nossa CW, et al. Inflammation and intestinal metaplasia of the distal esophagus are associated with alterations in the microbiome. Gastroenterology 2009;137(2):588–97.

37. Yang L, Francois F, Pei Z. Molecular pathways: pathogenesis and clinical implications of microbiome alteration in esophagitis and Barrett esophagus. Clin Cancer Res 2012;18(8):2138–44.

38. Fan YP, Chakder S, Gao F, et al. Inducible and neuronal nitric oxide synthase involvement in lipopolysaccharide-induced sphincteric dysfunction. Am J Physiol Gastrointest Liver Physiol 2001;280(1):G32–42.

39. Calatayud S, Garcia-Zaragoza E, Hernandez C, et al. Downregulation of nNOS and synthesis of PGs associated with endotoxin-induced delay in gastric emptying. Am J Physiol Gastrointest Liver Physiol 2002;283(6):G1360–7.

40. Liu N, Ando T, Ishiguro K, et al. Characterization of bacterial biota in the distal esophagus of Japanese patients with reflux esophagitis and Barrett's esophagus. BMC Infect Dis 2013;13:130.

41. Amir I, Konikoff FM, Oppenheim M, et al. Gastric microbiota is altered in oesophagitis and Barrett's oesophagus and further modified by proton pump inhibitors. Environ Microbiol 2013. http://dx.doi.org/10.1111/1462-2920.12285.

42. Rajilic-Stojanovic M, Biagi E, Heilig HG, et al. Global and deep molecular analysis of microbiota signatures in fecal samples from patients with irritable bowel syndrome. Gastroenterology 2011;141(5):1792–801.

43. Wang C, Yuan Y, Hunt RH. *Helicobacter pylori* infection and Barrett's esophagus: a systematic review and meta-analysis. Am J Gastroenterol 2009; 104(2):492–500 [quiz: 491, 501].

44. Rokkas T, Pistiolas D, Sechopoulos P, et al. Relationship between *Helicobacter pylori* infection and esophageal neoplasia: a meta-analysis. Clin Gastroenterol Hepatol 2007;5(12):1413–7, 1417.e1–2.

45. Fischbach LA, Graham DY, Kramer JR, et al. Association between *Helicobacter pylori* and Barrett's esophagus: a case-control study. Am J Gastroenterol 2014; 109(3):357–68.

46. Iwahi T, Satoh H, Nakao M, et al. Lansoprazole, a novel benzimidazole proton pump inhibitor, and its related compounds have selective activity against *Helicobacter pylori*. Antimicrob Agents Chemother 1991;35(3):490–6.

47. Chey WD, Wong BC, Practice Parameters Committee of the American College of Gastroenterology. American College of Gastroenterology guideline on the management of *Helicobacter pylori* infection. Am J Gastroenterol 2007;102(8): 1808–25.

48. Andersson AF, Lindberg M, Jakobsson H, et al. Comparative analysis of human gut microbiota by barcoded pyrosequencing. PLoS One 2008;3(7):e2836.

49. Sanduleanu S, Jonkers D, De Bruine A, et al. Non-*Helicobacter pylori* bacterial flora during acid-suppressive therapy: differential findings in gastric juice and gastric mucosa. Aliment Pharmacol Ther 2001;15(3):379–88.

50. Labenz J, Tillenburg B, Peitz U, et al. *Helicobacter pylori* augments the pH-increasing effect of omeprazole in patients with duodenal ulcer. Gastroenterology 1996;110(3):725–32.

51. Engstrand L, Lindberg M. *Helicobacter pylori* and the gastric microbiota. Best Pract Res Clin Gastroenterol 2013;27(1):39–45.

52. Zilberstein B, Quintanilha AG, Santos MA, et al. Digestive tract microbiota in healthy volunteers. Clinics (Sao Paulo) 2007;62(1):47–54.

53. Li XX, Wong GL, To KF, et al. Bacterial microbiota profiling in gastritis without *Helicobacter pylori* infection or non-steroidal anti-inflammatory drug use. PLoS One 2009;4(11):e7985.
54. Cover TL, Blaser MJ. *Helicobacter pylori* in health and disease. Gastroenterology 2009;136(6):1863–73.
55. Pereira SP, Gainsborough N, Dowling RH. Drug-induced hypochlorhydria causes high duodenal bacterial counts in the elderly. Aliment Pharmacol Ther 1998;12(1):99–104.
56. Houghton J, Wang TC. *Helicobacter pylori* and gastric cancer: a new paradigm for inflammation-associated epithelial cancers. Gastroenterology 2005;128(6):1567–78.
57. IARC working group on the evaluation of carcinogenic risks to humans: some industrial chemicals. Lyon, 15-22 February 1994. IARC Monogr Eval Carcinog Risks Hum 1994;60:1–560.
58. Wong BC, Lam SK, Wong WM, et al. *Helicobacter pylori* eradication to prevent gastric cancer in a high-risk region of China: a randomized controlled trial. JAMA 2004;291(2):187–94.
59. Ma JL, Zhang L, Brown LM, et al. Fifteen-year effects of *Helicobacter pylori*, garlic, and vitamin treatments on gastric cancer incidence and mortality. J Natl Cancer Inst 2012;104(6):488–92.
60. Malfertheiner P, Megraud F, O'Morain CA, et al. Management of *Helicobacter pylori* infection–the Maastricht IV/Florence Consensus Report. Gut 2012;61(5):646–64.
61. Liu WZ, Xie Y, Cheng H, et al. Fourth Chinese National Consensus Report on the management of *Helicobacter pylori* infection. J Dig Dis 2013;14(5):211–21.
62. Dicksved J, Lindberg M, Rosenquist M, et al. Molecular characterization of the stomach microbiota in patients with gastric cancer and in controls. J Med Microbiol 2009;58(Pt 4):509–16.
63. Tan MP, Kaparakis M, Galic M, et al. Chronic *Helicobacter pylori* infection does not significantly alter the microbiota of the murine stomach. Appl Environ Microbiol 2007;73(3):1010–3.
64. Wang TC, Dangler CA, Chen D, et al. Synergistic interaction between hypergastrinemia and *Helicobacter* infection in a mouse model of gastric cancer. Gastroenterology 2000;118(1):36–47.
65. Lofgren JL, Whary MT, Ge Z, et al. Lack of commensal flora in *Helicobacter pylori*-infected INS-GAS mice reduces gastritis and delays intraepithelial neoplasia. Gastroenterology 2011;140(1):210–20.
66. Lertpiriyapong K, Whary MT, Muthupalani S, et al. Gastric colonisation with a restricted commensal microbiota replicates the promotion of neoplastic lesions by diverse intestinal microbiota in the *Helicobacter pylori* INS-GAS mouse model of gastric carcinogenesis. Gut 2014;63(1):54–63.
67. Klinkenberg-Knol EC, Nelis F, Dent J, et al. Long-term omeprazole treatment in resistant gastroesophageal reflux disease: efficacy, safety, and influence on gastric mucosa. Gastroenterology 2000;118(4):661–9.
68. Lombardo L, Foti M, Ruggia O, et al. Increased incidence of small intestinal bacterial overgrowth during proton pump inhibitor therapy. Clin Gastroenterol Hepatol 2010;8(6):504–8.
69. Pyleris E, Giamarellos-Bourboulis EJ, Tzivras D, et al. The prevalence of overgrowth by aerobic bacteria in the small intestine by small bowel culture: relationship with irritable bowel syndrome. Dig Dis Sci 2012;57(5):1321–9.

70. Lo WK, Chan WW. Proton pump inhibitor use and the risk of small intestinal bacterial overgrowth: a meta-analysis. Clin Gastroenterol Hepatol 2013;11(5):483–90.
71. Bures J, Cyrany J, Kohoutova D, et al. Small intestinal bacterial overgrowth syndrome. World J Gastroenterol 2010;16(24):2978–90.
72. Williams C, McColl KE. Review article: proton pump inhibitors and bacterial overgrowth. Aliment Pharmacol Ther 2006;23(1):3–10.
73. Wallace JL, Syer S, Denou E, et al. Proton pump inhibitors exacerbate NSAID-induced small intestinal injury by inducing dysbiosis. Gastroenterology 2011;141(4):1314–22, 1322.e1–5.
74. Nadal I, Donat E, Ribes-Koninckx C, et al. Imbalance in the composition of the duodenal microbiota of children with coeliac disease. J Med Microbiol 2007; 56(Pt 12):1669–74.
75. Lebwohl B, Spechler SJ, Wang TC, et al. Use of proton pump inhibitors and subsequent risk of celiac disease. Dig Liver Dis 2014;46(1):36–40.
76. Lebwohl B, Blaser MJ, Ludvigsson JF, et al. Decreased risk of celiac disease in patients with *Helicobacter pylori* colonization. Am J Epidemiol 2013;178(12): 1721–30.
77. Robinson K, Kenefeck R, Pidgeon EL, et al. *Helicobacter pylori*-induced peptic ulcer disease is associated with inadequate regulatory T cell responses. Gut 2008;57(10):1375–85.
78. Walter J, Ley R. The human gut microbiome: ecology and recent evolutionary changes. Annu Rev Microbiol 2011;65:411–29.
79. Rawls JF, Mahowald MA, Ley RE, et al. Reciprocal gut microbiota transplants from zebrafish and mice to germ-free recipients reveal host habitat selection. Cell 2006;127(2):423–33.
80. Kwok CS, Arthur AK, Anibueze CI, et al. Risk of *Clostridium difficile* infection with acid suppressing drugs and antibiotics: meta-analysis. Am J Gastroenterol 2012;107(7):1011–9.
81. Janarthanan S, Ditah I, Adler DG, et al. *Clostridium difficile*-associated diarrhea and proton pump inhibitor therapy: a meta-analysis. Am J Gastroenterol 2012; 107(7):1001–10.
82. Dial S, Delaney JA, Barkun AN, et al. Use of gastric acid-suppressive agents and the risk of community-acquired *Clostridium difficile*-associated disease. JAMA 2005;294(23):2989–95.
83. Dial S, Delaney JA, Schneider V, et al. Proton pump inhibitor use and risk of community-acquired *Clostridium difficile*-associated disease defined by prescription for oral vancomycin therapy. CMAJ 2006;175(7):745–8.
84. Dial S, Alrasadi K, Manoukian C, et al. Risk of *Clostridium difficile* diarrhea among hospital inpatients prescribed proton pump inhibitors: cohort and case-control studies. CMAJ 2004;171(1):33–8.
85. Buendgens L, Bruensing J, Matthes M, et al. Administration of proton pump inhibitors in critically ill medical patients is associated with increased risk of developing *Clostridium difficile*-associated diarrhea. J Crit Care 2014;29:696.e11–5.
86. Chitnis AS, Holzbauer SM, Belflower RM, et al. Epidemiology of community-associated *Clostridium difficile* infection, 2009 through 2011. JAMA Intern Med 2013;173(14):1359–67.
87. Rao A, Jump RL, Pultz NJ, et al. In vitro killing of nosocomial pathogens by acid and acidified nitrite. Antimicrob Agents Chemother 2006;50(11):3901–4.
88. Wilson KH, Sheagren JN, Freter R. Population dynamics of ingested *Clostridium difficile* in the gastrointestinal tract of the Syrian hamster. J Infect Dis 1985; 151(2):355–61.

89. Kelly CP, LaMont JT. *Clostridium difficile*–more difficult than ever. N Engl J Med 2008;359(18):1932–40.
90. De La Cochetiere MF, Durand T, Lepage P, et al. Resilience of the dominant human fecal microbiota upon short-course antibiotic challenge. J Clin Microbiol 2005;43(11):5588–92.
91. Yu YH, Han DS, Choi EY, et al. Is use of PPIs related to increased intraepithelial lymphocytes in the colon? Dig Dis Sci 2012;57(10):2669–74.
92. Poullis A, Foster R, Mendall MA, et al. Proton pump inhibitors are associated with elevation of faecal calprotectin and may affect specificity. Eur J Gastroenterol Hepatol 2003;15(5):573–4 [author reply: 574].
93. Rechkemmer G, Frizzell RA, Halm DR. Active potassium transport across guinea-pig distal colon: action of secretagogues. J Physiol 1996;493(Pt 2): 485–502.
94. Freedberg DE, Salmasian H, Friedman C, et al. Proton pump inhibitors and risk for recurrent *Clostridium difficile* infection among inpatients. Am J Gastroenterol 2013;108(11):1794–801.
95. Linsky A, Gupta K, Lawler EV, et al. Proton pump inhibitors and risk for recurrent *Clostridium difficile* infection. Arch Intern Med 2010;170(9):772–8.
96. Manges AR, Labbe A, Loo VG, et al. Comparative metagenomic study of alterations to the intestinal microbiota and risk of nosocomial *Clostridum difficile*-associated disease. J Infect Dis 2010;202(12):1877–84.
97. Vincent C, Stephens DA, Loo VG, et al. Reductions in intestinal Clostridiales precede the development of nosocomial *Clostridium difficile* infection. Microbiome 2013;1(1):18.
98. Jakobsson HE, Jernberg C, Andersson AF, et al. Short-term antibiotic treatment has differing long-term impacts on the human throat and gut microbiome. PLoS One 2010;5(3):e9836.
99. Garcia-Mazcorro JF, Suchodolski JS, Jones KR, et al. Effect of the proton pump inhibitor omeprazole on the gastrointestinal bacterial microbiota of healthy dogs. FEMS Microbiol Ecol 2012;80(3):624–36.
100. Kanno T, Matsuki T, Oka M, et al. Gastric acid reduction leads to an alteration in lower intestinal microflora. Biochem Biophys Res Commun 2009;381(4):666–70.

Review of the Emerging Treatment of *Clostridium difficile* Infection with Fecal Microbiota Transplantation and Insights into Future Challenges

 CrossMark

Zain Kassam, MD, MPH, FRCPC[a], Christine H. Lee, MD, FRCPC[b,c,d],
Richard H. Hunt, MB, FRCP, FRCPEd, FRCPC, MACG, MWGO[e,f,*]

KEYWORDS

- *Clostridium difficile* • Health care–associated infections
- Fecal microbiota transplantation • Treatment

KEY POINTS

- *Clostridium difficile* infection (CDI) is one of the most common health care–associated infections in the United States, and there is concern regarding the emergence of community-acquired CDI.
- Currently, there are no standardized methods to prepare or deliver the fecal microbiota transplantation (FMT). Various methods are used to prepare the FMT, which is usually administered via nasogastric tube, colonoscopy, or by enema.
- Several clinical trials are underway to assess the true efficacy and safety of FMT for CDI. These trials include CDI studies assessing FMT via colonoscopy and frozen encapsulation, fresh versus frozen-and-thawed FMT by enema, FMT compared with a vancomycin taper, and FMT in the pediatric population.

[a] Department of Biological Engineering, Massachusetts Institute of Technology, 777 Massachusetts Avenue, 56-651, Cambridge, MA 02139, USA; [b] Division of Infectious Diseases, Department of Medicine, McMaster University, 1280 Main Street West, Hamilton, Ontario L8S 4K1, Canada; [c] Department of Pathology and Molecular Medicine, McMaster University, 1280 Main Street West, Hamilton, Ontario L8S 4L8, Canada; [d] Hamilton Regional Laboratory Medicine Program, 50 Charlton Avenue, Hamilton, Ontario L8N 4A6, Canada; [e] Division of Gastroenterology, Department of Medicine, McMaster University Health Science Centre, McMaster University, Room 3V3, 1280 Main Street West, Hamilton, Ontario L8S 4K1, Canada; [f] Farncombe Family Digestive Health Research Institute, Health Sciences Centre, Rm 3N4, 1280 Main Street West, Hamilton, Ontario L8S 4K1, Canada
* Corresponding author. Division of Gastroenterology, McMaster University Health Science Centre, Room 3V3, 1280 Main Street West, Hamilton, Ontario L8S 4K1, Canada.
E-mail address: huntr@mcmaster.ca

Clin Lab Med 34 (2014) 787–798
http://dx.doi.org/10.1016/j.cll.2014.08.007
0272-2712/14/$ – see front matter © 2014 Elsevier Inc. All rights reserved.

INTRODUCTION

Clostridium difficile infection (CDI) is one of the most common health care–associated infections in the United States, and there is concern regarding the emergence of community-acquired CDI.[1,2] CDI is associated with a spectrum of symptoms ranging from diarrhea to abdominal pain, and severe infections may lead to toxic megacolon and death. The clinical burden of CDI is significant. In the United States, the incidence of CDI doubled between 2000 and 2005 (5.5 cases per 10,000 vs 11.2 cases per 10,000 inpatient hospitalizations).[3] In Canada, 4.6 cases per 1000 patient admissions were reported in a national prospective surveillance study, and a recent study of 34 European countries suggested a weighted mean rate of 4.1 CDI cases per 10,000 patient-days per hospital.[4,5] CDI is also an evolving public health threat in low-income countries.[6] In addition to the increase in CDI incidence, the emergence of the hypervirulent and hypertransmissible North American pulse-field type 1/polymerase chain reaction (PCR) ribotype 027 (NAP1/027) strain has been associated with an increase in disease severity. A systematic review, capturing data from 11 European countries, suggests that CDI mortality rates more than doubled between the years 1999 and 2004. Rates continue to increase, and mortality is reported to be as high as 42% in some high-risk patient populations.[7] Canadian data also support the increase in attributable mortality. Surveillance data show an increase of approximately 4-fold between 1997 and 2005 (1.5% vs 5.7%).[4] The associated economic burden of CDI is substantial. Nosocomial CDI increases the cost of an otherwise matched hospitalization by 4-fold, translating to a reported cost of up to $4.8 billion per year in the United States.[8–10]

Although CDI antibiotic susceptibility testing is not routinely performed in clinical laboratories, there is growing clinical concern regarding microbial resistance and suboptimal efficacy of the standard antibiotic treatment. Since 2000, the failure rates of metronidazole, the recommended first-line treatment of mild to moderate CDI, have increased from 2.5% to more than 18.0%.[11] Other reports from Canada, the United Kingdom, and Spain have also documented resistance to metronidazole and reduced susceptibility to vancomycin in CDI.[12–14] However, the incidence of recurrent CDI following antibiotic treatment with metronidazole, vancomycin, or fidaxomicin continues to increase and has become a major challenge.[15–18] After 2 or more episodes of recurrence, the risk of subsequent recurrence has been reported to exceed 60% with antibiotic treatment.[16,19,20]

Given the shortcomings of antibiotic therapy, particularly in patients with recurrent CDI, alternative approaches have been explored for those who have failed standard antibiotic treatment.[15] One such therapy, fecal microbiota transplantation (FMT), has seen the growing scientific and public acceptance as a possible option in those who have failed standard treatments, in the hope of preventing hospitalization or colectomy. The hypothesized mechanism that underpins recurrent CDI is a lack of colonic microbial diversity; FMT aims to restore colonization resistance, reestablish diversity, and facilitate microbial homeostasis in order to protect against toxigenic CDI.[21–23]

The concept of FMT is not new and dates back to the Dong-Jin dynasty, fourth century China, where Ge Hong reported the oral ingestion of a human fecal suspension to resolve severe diarrhea.[24] Clinical cure rates with FMT in the modern era for the treatment of recurrent CDI are reported as approximately 90%.[25–28] These reports have revived interest in FMT, leading to an exponential increase in FMT publications and registered clinical trials over the last 5 years.[29]

FECAL MICROBIOTA TRANSPLANTATION EFFICACY IN *CLOSTRIDIUM DIFFICILE*

Despite the publication of an array of case reports and case series, until recently there has been a paucity of robust methodological studies evaluating FMT in CDI. Several systematic reviews have attempted to summarize the observational data, but there were intrinsic methodological limitations. These limitations were inclusion of unpublished data; an absence of an a priori minimum sample size threshold required to minimize the possibility of overestimating the treatment effect, given the inherent bias of case reports and small case series; and the omission of quality appraisal metrics, which are necessary when the evidence is of low quality on the hierarchy of evidence.[26–28] Recently, a more methodologically robust systematic review and meta-analysis was conducted that addressed the limitations of previous systematic reviews.[25] This review identified 11 studies with a total of 273 patients with CDI who were nonresponsive to standard antibiotics and treated with FMT. Of the patients, 89% experienced clinical resolution (95% confidence interval: 84%–93%).[25] A recent update using an identical methodological framework was conducted and yielded 5 additional case series.[30] Overall, the updated review identified 16 case series with a total of 526 patients with CDI who were not responding to standard antibiotics and treated with FMT. Of the patients, 88% experienced clinical resolution (95% confidence interval: 83%–92%), with cure rates ranging from 69% to 100%.[30] Given the dynamic development of the microbiome in the pediatric population, questions have been raised about the responsiveness of FMT in children.[31] In a recent systematic review, it seems that 5 out of 6 children with CDI, nonresponsive to standard antibiotics, responded to FMT.[28] These data must be interpreted with caution because of the small sample size and given that they were derived from case reports and, therefore, subject to overestimating the treatment effect.

The first randomized controlled trial for FMT in recurrent CDI following vancomycin therapy was reported by van Nood and colleagues[32]; the study was stopped early, at interim analysis, for benefit. Although methodologically imperfect, the trial results were nonetheless dramatic. FMT delivered by duodenal infusion yielded an 81% (13 of 16 patients) clinical cure rate, whereas the CDI resolution rate for vancomycin alone was only 31% (4 of 13 patients) and 23% (3 of 13 patients) for vancomycin, after bowel lavage (P<.001 for both comparisons with the FMT group). The clinical cure rate in the FMT arm increased to 94% when those who underwent a second FMT were included in the analysis.[32]

A subgroup analysis of a systematic review and meta-analysis suggested that FMT delivered by colonoscopy/enema (91% clinical success; 95% confidence interval: 86%–95%) led to higher clinical resolution rates than upper gastrointestinal delivery (82% clinical success; 95% confidence interval: 69%–90%) (proportion difference 9.1%, P<.05).[25] Building on this hypothesis, a small (n = 20) randomized controlled trial was conducted. Youngster and colleagues[33] conducted a randomized, controlled, open-label trial comparing nasogastric versus colonoscopic FMT delivery using a frozen fecal suspension from a healthy, screened, and unrelated donor. Although this study was underpowered to detect a meaningful difference between treatment arms, a single FMT administered by colonoscopy yielded an 80% (8 of 10 patients) clinical cure rate, whereas the CDI resolution rate with nasogastric administration was 60% (6 of 10 patients). Five patients who did not achieve a clinical cure were retreated by nasogastric administration for a total of 100% (10 of 10 patients) clinical cure in the colonoscopy arm and 80% (8 of 10 patients) in the nasogastric administration arm. No patients relapsed clinically at the 8-week follow-up.[33]

The clinical efficacy of FMT is complemented by its economic benefit. In a decision analysis assessing the cost-effectiveness of competing strategies for the management of recurrent CDI, FMT by colonoscopy was found favorable.[34] FMT by colonoscopy had an incremental cost-effectiveness ratio of $17,016 relative to oral vancomycin. FMT by colonoscopy was much more cost-effective compared with metronidazole or fidaxomicin use.[34] There is an important methodological consideration in this study regarding the route of FMT delivery. The study obtained the CDI cure rate for FMT delivery by enema from a report that included predominantly inpatients (81%), which may be a surrogate for more serious disease, and NAP-1 was not tested.[35] In contrast, the 94.5% CDI cure rate described for FMT by colonoscopy delivery in the decision analysis was driven by a study that assessed largely outpatients (86%).[36] Accordingly, the reduced efficacy of enema compared with colonoscopy may not be caused by the mode of delivery but rather the patient population, in turn, impacting the results favoring FMT delivered by colonoscopy. Although head-to-head studies of the mode of delivery and dosing in standardized patient populations are warranted, enema may be the ideal first-line mode of delivery, when examining the totality of evidence, even if efficacy rates are slightly lower. Specifically, enema is more accessible and can be performed by any clinician in contrast to colonoscopy, which requires extensive resources and specialized personnel. Additionally, procedure-associated adverse events, such as perforation, are more common among patients undergoing colonoscopic delivery when compared with enema.[25,37]

FECAL MICROBIOTA TRANSPLANTATION AND ITS NEXUS WITH CLINICAL GUIDELINES

Given the scope of CDI and its multidisciplinary nature, evidence-based guidelines have been established by several organizations. These guidelines have included treatment approaches for recurrent CDI and more specific guidelines regarding FMT. The 2010 CDI clinical practice guidelines from the Society for Healthcare Epidemiology of America and the Infectious Diseases Society of America suggest vancomycin in a tapered and/or pulsed regimen for second CDI recurrence treatment (grade B-III). They find a third recurrence challenging and consider FMT as an option given the high degree of success in uncontrolled studies. However, they do not provide further insights beyond recommending donors be screened for transmissible agents and considerations be given for logistic issues, such as the route of administration.[38] The 2013 American College of Gastroenterology's CDI guidelines suggest consideration of FMT "if there is a third recurrence after a pulsed vancomycin regimen (conditional recommendation, moderate-quality evidence),"[39] although no specific recommendations regarding the delivery modality or donor type (directed vs universal donor) are given. The 2014 treatment guidance of the European Society of Clinical Microbiology and Infectious Diseases recommend oral vancomycin or fidaxomicin for nonsevere second (or later) recurrent CDI.[40] Moreover, they acknowledge that there are no prospective randomized controlled trials investigating the efficacy of fidaxomicin in patients with *multiple* recurrences of CDI. However, the American College of Gastroenterology does recommend FMT for treating multiple recurrent CDI (strength of recommendation: A, quality of evidence: I), although the guidelines are less clear on specific FMT recommendations.[40] Although there are American and Canadian FMT working groups that have published best practice reviews, there is still considerable heterogeneity in the mechanics of FMT.[25,41–43] For example, although the risk factors for infectious disease, gastrointestinal comorbidities, and the use of drugs, such as antibiotics or probiotics, that affect the microbiome are common exclusion criteria for stool donors, the presence of potentially microbiome-mediated medical conditions, such as donor neuro-psychiatric illness or obesity, is either omitted or poorly described.[44] The 2014 Canadian Association of Gastroenterology's position statement on FMT echoes the previous reports regarding the paucity of studies that have formally sought to evaluate the adverse effects prospectively, which contributes to underreporting.[25,30] The Canadian Association of Gastroenterology called for an emphasis on safety and counseling for FMT patients concerning the known and unknown risks, which is appropriate for all patients undergoing this procedure. Although there have been plausible adverse events related to the mode of FMT delivery, case series data have recently highlighted concerns over norovirus and the possibility of autoimmune disease transmission, strengthening the need to follow FMT recipients and established long-term safety registries.[45–47]

TECHNICAL REVIEW

Currently, there are no standardized methods to prepare or deliver the FMT. Various methods are used to prepare the FMT, which is usually administered via nasogastric tube, colonoscopy, or by enema.[32,35,36,43,48–50] The best means to prepare, the ideal volume to use, and the optimal mode of delivery are yet to be defined. The following are important considerations before preparing the FMT. First, the transplant unit must ensure the availability of more than 1 reliable and fully screened donor. A comprehensive donor screening consisting of medical history and physical examination should be performed. Donors should be excluded when there is any history of autoimmune disease, active cancer, systemic antibiotic use within the past 12 weeks, risk factors for underlying human immunodeficiency virus (HIV)/sexually transmitted infections, prion disease, gastrointestinal disease, or family history of colonic cancer. The approach to donor screening by laboratory testing is summarized in **Table 1** and well described by Bakken and colleagues.[41] Second, the stool samples should be prepared in a laboratory with a level-2 biological safety cabinet (BSC) because the stools are designated as a level-2 biohazard specimen. It is essential that the FMT manufacturing laboratory meets the standards of the clinical laboratory accreditation program to ensure the safety of FMT.[41,42]

With regard to the actual processing of stool samples to manufacture FMT, stool is mixed with a diluent: bottled water,[36,51] preservative-free normal saline,[27,52] or milk.[53] Some centers use a homogenizer or a standard household[49] or a commercial-grade blender[54] to emulsify, whereas others use manual manipulation to break down stool samples.[36,51,55] For manual preparation of stool samples, the stool and diluent are mixed directly in the sample collection container, fitted with an airtight lid, and either shaken vigorously or mixed with a disposable plastic or wooden spatula. The

Table 1
Donor screening laboratory testing

Specimen	Pathogen	Laboratory Tests
Serum	HAV	HAV IgM and IgG
	HBV	HB surface antigen; antibody to HB core
	HCV	HCV antibody
	HIV 1 & 2	EIA
	HTLV 1 & II	EIA
	Treponema pallidum	Syphilis IgG and rapid plasma reagin
Stool	*Clostridium difficile* toxins	PCR or combined *Clostridium difficile* common antigen and toxin detection EIA
	Enteric bacteria	Stool culture
	Ova and parasites	Light microscopy and EIA for *Giardia, Cryptosporidium*
	Helicobacter pylori antigen (if used for nasogastric delivery)	EIA

Abbreviations: EIA, enzyme immunoassay; HAV, hepatitis A virus; HB, hepatitis B; HBV, hepatitis B virus; HCV, hepatitis C virus; HTLV, human T-lymphocyte virus; IgG, immunoglobulin G; IgM, immunoglobulin M.

advantages of using manual techniques are as follows: it requires no maintenance or disinfection of equipment and low cost. There is minimal to no potential for aerosolization or injury to the operator. The sample preparation time takes less than 10 minutes. The advantage of using a blender or a homogenizer is that the mixture is devoid of particulates. The disadvantages of using a blender are the need to disinfect after each use and a greater potential for generating aerosols compared with the manual processing.

Approximately 50 g of stool sample, maintained at 5°C to 8°C, should be in the laboratory within 5 hours of collection. Using a hood or BSC, the stool sample is mixed with 300 mL of either preservative-free saline or commercially available bottled drinking water or milk. The mixture can be emulsified using an electric blender, homogenizer, or manually.[36,49,54] In order to minimize solid particles from clogging up the colonoscope channel or the tip of a syringe, the mixture is filtered using 4 × 4 in gauze,[46,50,51] coffee filters,[48] or a stainless steel laboratory sieve.[54] It is important to process the stool within 1 hour of receipt to avoid excess exposure to ambient temperature and oxygen; in order to optimize the survival of anaerobes, one center processed the FMT under nitrogen gas.[54] One study reported preparation of stool for FMT in an anaerobic chamber.[56] Following the filtration, the infusate is aspirated into a 60-mL syringe and administered using the same syringe as the enema or via colonoscopy or nasogastric route. Two centers have stored fecal suspension at −80°C for 1 to 8 weeks and thawed in ice or a 37°C bath before FMT.[33,54]

More recently, different strategies have been developed to administer bacteria for the treatment of recurrent CDI. One is a synthetic stool mixture developed by a group of researchers in Ontario, Canada, which was infused at colonoscopy into the colon of 2 patients with recurrent CDI.[57] The synthetic stool was created using 33 different strains of intestinal bacteria cultured in strict anaerobic conditions from a single healthy donor and mixed in 100 mL of 0.9% sodium chloride to an approximate concentration of 3.5×10^9 colony-forming units per millimeter. This mixture was infused at colonoscopy into the colon of the 2 patients with recurrent CDI who were also infected with the ribotype 078 strain. At the 6-month follow-up, there was no evidence of recurrent disease in either patient.[57]

A second group of investigators from Alberta, Canada have developed oral bacterial capsules to provide to patients who could not retain an enema or tolerate a jejunal catheter. Freshly collected fecal samples were centrifuged following prereduction in phosphate buffered saline (PBS) to produce pellets of "intestinal microbes." The sediment was resuspended in a minimal volume of PBS and pipetted into gelatin capsules, which were re-encapsulated to ensure the delivery of viable bacteria into the colon. Twenty-seven patients with recurrent CDI ingested between 24 and 34 microbe-containing double overencapsulated gelatin capsules. All patients had resolution of CDI, and there were no adverse events in the follow-up.[58]

FUTURE DIRECTIONS OF FECAL MICROBIOTA TRANSPLANTATION

Several clinical trials are underway to assess the true efficacy and safety of FMT for CDI. These trials include CDI studies assessing FMT via colonoscopy[59] and frozen encapsulation,[60] fresh versus frozen-and-thawed FMT by enema,[61] FMT compared with a vancomycin taper,[62] and FMT in the pediatric population.[63] The results of these trials may shed light with regard to the best method to prepare and deliver FMT. In contrast to FMT whereby a complete microbial ecosystem is restored, there has been increasing interest in a specific, defined microbial strains approach to treat CDI.[64] Although a synthetic stool seems promising, there may be barriers related to the costs associated with the equipment and the labor-intensive manufacturing process. Patients and clinicians are eager to move forward with an oral bacterial capsule approach. However, this approach will likely be refined to a narrow patient population who are able to tolerate swallowing 20 to 40 capsules and do not have esophageal disease or dysphagia issues or are at risk for oropharyngeal aspiration. Overall, FMT delivered by enema seems to be the least invasive, well tolerated by patients, has a low cost, and can be administered by any health care provider with minimal training. Therefore, FMT by enema may become the most widely practiced method for initial FMT.

FECAL MICROBIOTA TRANSPLANTATION: CURRENT REGULATORY LANDSCAPE

In May 2013, the US Food and Drug Administration (FDA) delivered a public message that it would regulate human stool as a biological product and an investigational drug, in turn, requiring physicians to complete a laborious, 12- to 18-month investigational new drug (IND) application before performing FMT in any patient.[29,65] The FDA rationalized this requirement as a way to promote overall safer FMT, standardize therapy, and empower commercial development. At a public workshop jointly sponsored by the FDA and the National Institutes of Health, patients, physicians, and scientists expressed significant concerns that the IND process may deter physicians from providing FMT to patients and that this, in turn, might encourage patients to seek home FMTs using unscreened stools. Subsequently, the FDA revised its position and, currently, has opted to "exercise enforcement discretion," enabling physicians to provide FMTs specifically to patients with CDI who are not responding to standard treatments following informed consent, however, without an IND approval.[29,65]

Under the FDA exemption, the concept of a stool bank, analogous to blood banks, has emerged to assist clinicians in delivering FMT expeditiously. At least 2 large academic hospitals have established stool banks for their own patients: Massachusetts General Hospital and Emory University Hospital. A nonprofit organization, OpenBiome, has centralized and standardized the rigorous screening and preparation process. It provides screened and prepared stool, which is frozen and shipped to clinicians for FMT delivery after appropriate thawing or stored in $-20°C$ or $-80°C$ freezer for downstream clinical use. As the screening costs are amortized over many samples from each donor, the screening costs per treatment are $250, a marginal expense compared with the directed donor approach. To date, OpenBiome has delivered more than 600 treatment stools to more than 60 US hospitals in 26 states. OpenBiome is also working on a study designed to examine the long-term safety of FMT in order to assist the FDA in guiding the regulatory trajectory of FMT.[29,66]

Recently, the FDA posted a *draft* of a new guidance, which states: "[The] FDA intends to exercise this discretion provided that [the donated stool] is obtained from a donor known to either the patient or to the licensed health care provider treating the patient."[67] The criteria for the "known to" donor have not been established, and there has been considerable public concern voiced in opposition of this draft for an array of reasons. Importantly, the draft has not been made an official guidance; it is unclear if that will occur.[67] Accordingly, stool banks, such as OpenBiome and others, have been able to continue to provide FMT.

Given that the active ingredients in stool are not known and there is significant heterogeneity between stool samples, FMT does not fit well into the standard definition of a drug. Therefore, FMT may best be regulated as a human tissue or tissuelike product, such as blood, which requires rigorous FDA-approved screening processes. This guidance currently presents a challenge because US laws exclude products that are excreted from the body, thus disqualifying stool. An exception has been made for semen; many are advocating a similar exception for stool[29] to enable FMT to be safe, accessible, and affordable.

REFERENCES

1. Magill SS, Edwards JR, Bamberg W, et al. Multistate point-prevalence survey of health care-associated infections. N Engl J Med 2014;370(13):1198–208.
2. Collins C, Ayturk M, Flahive J. Epidemiology and outcomes of community-acquired Clostridium difficile infections in Medicare beneficiaries. J Am Coll Surg 2014;218(6):1141–8.
3. Zilberberg M, Shorr A, Kollef M. Increase in adult Clostridium difficile–related hospitalizations and case-fatality rate, United States, 2000–2005. Emerg Infect Dis 2008;14(6):929–31.
4. Gravel D, Miller M, Simor A, et al. Health care' associated Clostridium difficile infection in adults admitted to acute care hospitals in Canada: a Canadian noso-comial infection surveillance program study. Clin Infect Dis 2009;48(5):568–76. http://dx.doi.org/10.1086/596703.
5. Bauer MP, Notermans DW, van Benthem BH, et al. Clostridium difficile infection in Europe: a hospital-based survey. Lancet 2011;377(9759):63–73. http://dx.doi.org/10.1016/S0140-6736(10)61266-4.
6. Simango C, Uladi S. Detection of Clostridium difficile diarrhoea in Harare, Zimbabwe. Trans R Soc Trop Med Hyg 2014;108(6):354–7. http://dx.doi.org/10.1093/trstmh/tru042.
7. Wiegand PN, Nathwani D, Wilcox MH, et al. Clinical and economic burden of Clostridium difficile infection in Europe: a systematic review of health care-facility-acquired infection. J Hosp Infect 2012;81(1):1–14. http://dx.doi.org/10.1016/j.jhin.2012.02.004.
8. McGlone S, Bailey R, Zimmer S. The economic burden of Clostridium difficile. Clin Microbiol Infect 2012;18(3):282–9. http://dx.doi.org/10.1111/j.1469-0691.2011.03571.x.
9. Dubberke E, Olsen M. Burden of Clostridium difficile on the health care system. Clin Infect Dis 2012;55(Suppl 2):S88–92. http://dx.doi.org/10.1093/cid/cis335.
10. Vonberg R, Reichardt C, Behnke M. Cost of nosocomial Clostridium difficile-associated diarrhoea. J Hosp Infect 2008;70:15–20.
11. Kelly CP, Lamont JT. Clostridium difficile — more difficult than ever. N Engl J Med 2008;359:1932–40.
12. Lynch T, Chong P, Zhang J, et al. Characterization of a stable, metronidazole-resistant clostridium difficile clinical isolate. PLoS One 2013;8(1):e53757. http://dx.doi.org/10.1371/journal.pone.0053757.
13. Baines SD, O'Connor R, Freeman J, et al. Emergence of reduced susceptibility to metronidazole in Clostridium difficile. J Antimicrob Chemother 2008;62(5):1046–52. http://dx.doi.org/10.1093/jac/dkn313.
14. Peláez T, Alcalá L, Alonso R, et al. Reassessment of Clostridium difficile suscep-tibility to metronidazole and vancomycin. Antimicrob Agents Chemother 2002;46(6):1647–50. http://dx.doi.org/10.1128/AAC.46.6.1647.
15. O'Horo JC, Jindai K, Kunzer B, et al. Treatment of recurrent Clostridium difficile infection: a systematic review. Infection 2014;42(1):43–59. http://dx.doi.org/10.1007/s15010-013-0496-x.
16. Petrella LA, Sambol SP, Cheknis A, et al. Decreased cure and increased recur-rence rates for clostridium difficile infection caused by the epidemic C. difficile BI strain. Clin Infect Dis 2012;55(3):351–7. http://dx.doi.org/10.1093/cid/cis430.

17. Barbut F, Richard A, Hamadi K. Epidemiology of recurrences or reinfections of Clostridium difficile epidemiology of recurrences or reinfections of Clostridium difficile -associated diarrhea. J Clin Microbiol 2000;38(6):2386–8.
18. Louie TJ, Miller MA, Mullane KM, et al. Fidaxomicin versus vancomycin for Clostridium difficile infection. N Engl J Med 2011;364(5):422–31.
19. Pépin J, Saheb N, Coulombe MA, et al. Emergence of fluoroquinolones as the predominant risk factor for Clostridium difficile-associated diarrhea: a cohort study during an epidemic in Quebec. Clin Infect Dis 2005;41(9):1254–60.
20. McFarland LV, Elmer GW, Surawicz CM. Breaking the cycle: treatment strategies for 163 cases of recurrent Clostridium difficile disease. Am J Gastroenterol 2002;97(7):1769–75.
21. Song Y, Garg S, Girotra M, et al. Microbiota dynamics in patients treated with fecal microbiota transplantation for recurrent Clostridium difficile infection. PLoS One 2013;8(11):e81330. http://dx.doi.org/10.1371/journal.pone. 0081330.
22. Chang JY, Antonopoulos DA, Kalra A, et al. Decreased diversity of the fecal microbiome in recurrent Clostridium difficile-associated diarrhea. J Infect Dis 2008;197(3):435–8. http://dx.doi.org/10.1086/525047.
23. Khoruts A, Dicksved J, Jansson JK, et al. Khoruts 2010. J Clin Gastroenterol 2010;44(5):354–60.
24. Zhang F, Luo W, Shi Y, et al. Should we standardize the 1,700-year-old fecal microbiota transplantation? Am J Gastroenterol 2012;107(11):1755. http://dx.doi. org/10.1038/ajg.2012.251 [author reply: 1755–6].
25. Kassam Z, Lee CH, Yuan Y, et al. Fecal microbiota transplantation for Clostridium difficile infection: systematic review and meta-analysis. Am J Gastroenterol 2013;108(4):500–8. http://dx.doi.org/10.1038/ajg.2013.59.
26. Guo B, Harstall C, Louie T, et al. Systematic review: faecal transplantation for the treatment of Clostridium difficile-associated disease. Aliment Pharmacol Ther 2012;35(8):865–75. http://dx.doi.org/10.1111/j.1365-2036.2012.05033.x.
27. Gough E, Shaikh H, Manges AR. Systematic review of intestinal microbiota transplantation (fecal bacteriotherapy) for recurrent clostridium difficile infection. Clin Infect Dis 2011;53(10):994–1002. http://dx.doi.org/10.1093/cid/cir632.
28. Sha S, Liang J, Chen M, et al. Systematic review: faecal microbiota transplantation therapy for digestive and nondigestive disorders in adults and children. Aliment Pharmacol Ther 2014;39(10):1003–32. http://dx.doi.org/10.1111/apt. 12699.
29. Smith MB, Kelly C, Alm EJ. How to regulate faecal transplants. Nature 2014;506: 290–1.
30. Moayyedi P, Marshall JK, Yuan Y, et al. Canadian Association of Gastroenterology position statement: fecal microbiota transplant therapy. Can J Gastroenterol 2014;28(2):1–3.
31. Kassam Z, Murray TS. Navigating the pediatric microbiome: emerging evidence and clinical implications. Curr Pediatr Rep 2014;2(2):93–101. http://dx.doi.org/ 10.1007/s40124-014-0040-1.
32. Van Nood E, Vrieze A, Nieuwdorp M, et al. Duodenal infusion of donor feces for recurrent Clostridium difficile. N Engl J Med 2013;368(5):407–15. http://dx.doi. org/10.1056/NEJMoa1205037.
33. Youngster I, Sauk J, Pindar C, et al. Fecal microbiota transplant for relapsing Clostridium difficile infection using a frozen inoculum from unrelated donors: a randomized, open-label, controlled pilot study. Clin Infect Dis 2014;58(11): 1–8. http://dx.doi.org/10.1093/cid/ciu135.

34. Konijeti GG, Sauk J, Shrime MG, et al. Cost-effectiveness of competing strategies for management of recurrent Clostridium difficile infection: a decision analysis. Clin Infect Dis 2014;58(11):1–8. http://dx.doi.org/10.1093/cid/ciu128.

35. Kassam Z, Hundal R, Marshall J, et al. Fecal transplant via retention enema for refractory or recurrent clostridium difficile infection. Arch Intern Med 2012; 172(2):2012–4.

36. Mattila E, Uusitalo-Seppälä R, Wuorela M, et al. Fecal transplantation, through colonoscopy, is effective therapy for recurrent Clostridium difficile infection. Gastroenterology 2012;142(3):490–6. http://dx.doi.org/10.1053/j.gastro.2011. 11.037.

37. Kelly CR, Ihunnah C, Fischer M, et al. Fecal microbiota transplant for treatment of Clostridium difficile infection in immunocompromised patients. Am J Gastroenterol 2014;109(7):1065–71. http://dx.doi.org/10.1038/ajg.2014.133.

38. Cohen SH, Gerding DN, Johnson S, et al. Clinical practice guidelines for Clostridium difficile infection in adults: 2010 update by the society for health care epidemiology of America (SHEA) and the infectious diseases society of America (IDSA). Infect Control Hosp Epidemiol 2010;31(5):431–55. http://dx.doi.org/10. 1086/651706.

39. Surawicz CM, Brandt LJ, Binion DG, et al. Guidelines for diagnosis, treatment, and prevention of Clostridium difficile infections. Am J Gastroenterol 2013; 108(4):478–98. http://dx.doi.org/10.1038/ajg.2013.4 [quiz: 499].

40. Debast SB, Bauer MP, Kuijper EJ. Comm. European Society of Clinical Microbiology and Infectious Diseases: update of the treatment guidance document for Clostridium difficile infection. Clin Microbiol Infect 2014;20(2):1–26.

41. Bakken JS, Borody T, Brandt LJ, et al. Treating Clostridium difficile infection with fecal microbiota transplantation. Clin Gastroenterol Hepatol 2011;9(12):1044–9. http://dx.doi.org/10.1016/j.cgh.2011.08.014.

42. Allen-Vercoe E, Reid G, Viner N, et al. A Canadian Working Group report on fecal microbial therapy: microbial ecosystems therapeutics. Can J Gastroenterol 2012;26(7):457–62.

43. Lee CH, Belanger JE, Kassam Z, et al. The outcome and long-term follow-up of 94 patients with recurrent and refractory Clostridium difficile infection using single to multiple fecal microbiota transplantation via retention enema. Eur J Clin Microbiol Infect Dis 2014;33:1425–8. http://dx.doi.org/10.1007/s10096-014-2088-9.

44. Collins SM, Kassam Z, Bercik P. The adoptive transfer of behavioral phenotype via the intestinal microbiota: experimental evidence and clinical implications. Curr Opin Microbiol 2013;16(3):240–5.

45. Schwartz M, Gluck M, Koon S. Norovirus gastroenteritis after fecal microbiota transplantation for treatment of Clostridium difficile infection despite asymptomatic donors and lack of sick contacts. Am J Gastroenterol 2013;108(8):1367. http://dx.doi.org/10.1038/ajg.2013.164.

46. Brandt LJ, Aroniadis OC, Mellow M, et al. Long-term follow-up of colonoscopic fecal microbiota transplant for recurrent Clostridium difficile infection. Am J Gastroenterol 2012;107(7):1079–87. http://dx.doi.org/10.1038/ajg.2012.60.

47. Kassam Z, Lee CH, Yuan Y, et al. Navigating long-term safety in fecal microbiota transplantation. Am J Gastroenterol 2013;108(9):1538. http://dx.doi.org/10. 1038/ajg.2013.214.

48. Aas J, Gessert CE, Bakken JS. Recurrent Clostridium difficile colitis: case series involving 18 patients treated with donor stool administered via a nasogastric tube. Clin Infect Dis 2003;36(5):580–5. http://dx.doi.org/10.1086/367657.

49. Silverman MS, Davis I, Pillai DR. Success of self-administered home fecal transplantation for chronic Clostridium difficile infection. Clin Gastroenterol Hepatol 2010;8(5):471–3. http://dx.doi.org/10.1016/j.cgh.2010.01.007.

50. Yoon SS, Brandt LJ. Treatment of refractory/recurrent C. difficile- associated disease by donated stool transplanted via colonoscopy: a case series of 12 patients. J Clin Gastroenterol 2010;44(8):562–6.

51. Kelly CR, de Leon L, Jasutkar N. Fecal microbiota transplantation for relapsing Clostridium difficile infection in 26 patients: methodology and results. J Clin Gastroenterol 2012;46(2):145–9. http://dx.doi.org/10.1097/MCG.0b013e318234570b.

52. Borody TJ, Warren EF, Leis SM, et al. Bacteriotherapy using fecal flora. J Clin Gastroenterol 2004;38(6):475–83. http://dx.doi.org/10.1097/01.mcg.0000128988.13808.dc.

53. Lund-Tønnesen S, Berstad A, Schreiner A, et al. Clostridium difficile-associated diarrhea treated with homologous feces. Tidsskr Nor Laegeforen 1998;118(17):1027–30.

54. Hamilton MJ, Weingarden AR, Sadowsky MJ, et al. Standardized frozen preparation for transplantation of fecal microbiota for recurrent Clostridium difficile infection. Am J Gastroenterol 2012;107(5):761–7. http://dx.doi.org/10.1038/ajg.2011.482.

55. Garborg K, Waagsbø B, Stallemo A, et al. Results of faecal donor instillation therapy for recurrent Clostridium difficile-associated diarrhoea. Scand J Infect Dis 2010;42(11–12):857–61. http://dx.doi.org/10.3109/00365548.2010.499541.

56. Schwan A, Sjolin S, Trottestam U, et al. Relapsing Clostridium difficile enterocolitis cured by rectal infusion of homologous faeces. Lancet 1983;2(8354):845.

57. Petrof EO, Gloor GB, Vanner SJ, et al. Stool substitute transplant therapy for the eradication of Clostridium difficile infection: "RePOOPulating" the gut. Microbiome 2013;1(1):3. http://dx.doi.org/10.1186/2049-2618-1-3.

58. Louie T, Cannon K, O'Grady H, et al. Fecal microbiome transplantation (FMT) via oral fecal microbial capsules for recurrent Clostridium difficile infection (rCDI). Abstract presented at The ID Week Conference. 2014.

59. Kelly C. Fecal transplant for relapsing C. Difficile infection. 2014. U.S. National Institutes of Health Trial Register. NCT Number 01703494. Available at: http://www.clinicaltrials.gov/ct2/show/NCT01703494?term=fecal+transplant & rank=4. Accessed July 14, 2014.

60. Hohmann EL. Fecal microbiota transplant for relapsing Clostridium difficile infection in adults and children using a frozen encapsulated inoculum. 2014. U.S. National Institutes of Health Trial Register. NCT Number NCT01914731. Available at: http://clinicaltrials.gov/ct2/show/NCT01914731?term=fecal&rank=17. Accessed July 14, 2014.

61. Lee C. Multi-centre trial of fresh vs frozen-and-thawed HBT (fecal transplant) for recurrent CDI. 2014. Available at: U.S. National Institutes of Health Trial Register. NCT Number 01398969. Available at: http://www.clinicaltrials.gov/ct2/show/NCT01398969?term=fecal+transplant & rank=2. Accessed July 14, 2014.

62. Hota S. Oral vancomycin followed by fecal transplant vs. tapering oral vancomycin. 2014. U.S. National Institutes of Health Trial Register. NCT Number 01226992. Available at: http://www.clinicaltrials.gov/ct2/show/NCT01226992?term=feca l+transplant & rank=1. Accessed July 12, 2014.

63. Gisser J. Fecal transplant for pediatric patients who have recurrent C-diff infection (FMT). 2014. Available at: U.S. National Institutes of Health Trial Register. NCT Number NCT02134392. Available at: http://clinicaltrials.gov/ct2/show/NCT02134392?term=gisser&rank=1. Accessed July 12, 2014.

64. Lawley TD, Clare S, Walker AW, et al. Targeted restoration of the intestinal microbiota with a simple, defined bacteriotherapy resolves relapsing Clostridium difficile disease in mice. PLoS Pathog 2012;8(10):e1002995. http://dx.doi.org/10.1371/journal.ppat.1002995.

65. Merenstein D, El-Nachef N, Lynch S. Fecal microbial therapy - promises and pitfalls. J Pediatr Gastroenterol Nutr 2014. http://dx.doi.org/10.1097/MPG.000000000000415.

66. Smith M, Kassam Z, Edelstein C, et al. OpenBiome. 2014. Available at: http://www.openbiome.org/. Accessed July, 2014.

67. FDA. Vaccine and Related Biological Product Guidances - draft guidance for industry: enforcement policy regarding investigational new drug requirements for use of fecal microbiota for transplantation to treat Clostridium difficile infection not responsive to standard therapies. 2014. Available at: http://www.fda.gov/BiologicsBloodVaccines/GuidanceComplianceRegulatoryInformation/Guidances/Vaccines/ucm387023.htm?source=govdelivery&utm_medium=email&utm_source=govdelivery. Accessed September 18, 2014.

Index

Note: Page numbers of article titles are in **boldface** type.

Clin Lab Med 34 (2014) 799–806
http://dx.doi.org/10.1016/S0272-2712(14)00092-4
0272-2712/14/$ – see front matter © 2014 Elsevier Inc. All rights reserved.

labmed.theclinics.com

United States Postal Service

Statement of Ownership, Management, and Circulation
(All Periodicals Publications Except Requestor Publications)

1. Publication Title	2. Publication Number	3. Filing Date
Clinics in Laboratory Medicine	0 1 2 - 9 6 0 0	9/14/14

4. Issue Frequency	5. Number of Issues Published Annually	6. Annual Subscription Price
Mar, Jun, Sep, Dec	4	$250.00

7. Complete Mailing Address of Known Office of Publication (Not printer) (Street, city, county, state, and ZIP+4®)

Elsevier Inc.
360 Park Avenue South
New York, NY 10010-1710

Contact Person
Stephen R. Bushing

Telephone (Include area code)
215-239-3688

8. Complete Mailing Address of Headquarters or General Business Office of Publisher (Not printer)

Elsevier Inc., 360 Park Avenue South, New York, NY 10010-1710

9. Full Names and Complete Mailing Addresses of Publisher, Editor, and Managing Editor (Do not leave blank)

Publisher (Name and complete mailing address)

Linda Belfus, Elsevier Inc., 1600 John F. Kennedy Blvd., Suite 1800, Philadelphia, PA 19103-2899

Editor (Name and complete mailing address)

Joanne Husovski, Elsevier Inc., 1600 John F. Kennedy Blvd., Suite 1800, Philadelphia, PA 19103-2899

Managing Editor (Name and complete mailing address)

Adrianne Brigido, Elsevier Inc, 1600 John F. Kennedy Blvd., Suite 1800, Philadelphia, PA 19103-2899

10. Owner (Do not leave blank. If the publication is owned by a corporation, give the name and address of the corporation immediately followed by the names and addresses of all stockholders owning or holding 1 percent or more of the total amount of stock. If not owned by a corporation, give the names and addresses of the individual owners. If owned by a partnership or other unincorporated firm, give its name and address as well as those of each individual owner. If the publication is published by a nonprofit organization, give its name and address.)

Full Name	Complete Mailing Address
Wholly owned subsidiary of	1600 John F. Kennedy Blvd., Ste. 1800
Reed/Elsevier, US holdings	Philadelphia, PA 19103-2899

11. Known Bondholders, Mortgagees, and Other Security Holders Owning or Holding 1 Percent or More of Total Amount of Bonds, Mortgages, or Other Securities. If none, check box ☒ None

Full Name	Complete Mailing Address
N/A	

12. Tax Status (For completion by nonprofit organizations authorized to mail at nonprofit rates) (Check one)
The purpose, function, and nonprofit status of this organization and the exempt status for federal income tax purposes:
☐ Has Not Changed During Preceding 12 Months
☐ Has Changed During Preceding 12 Months (Publisher must submit explanation of change with this statement)

PS Form 3526, August 2012 (Page 1 of 3 (Instructions Page 3)) PSN 7530-01-000-9931 PRIVACY NOTICE: See our Privacy policy in www.usps.com

---

13. Publication Title	14. Issue Date for Circulation Data Below
Clinics in Laboratory Medicine	June 2014

15. Extent and Nature of Circulation		Average No. Copies Each Issue During Preceding 12 Months	No. Copies of Single Issue Published Nearest to Filing Date
a. Total Number of Copies (Net press run)		328	320
b. Paid Circulation (By Mail and Outside the Mail)	(1) Mailed Outside-County Paid Subscriptions Stated on PS Form 3541 (Include paid distribution above nominal rate, advertiser's proof copies, and exchange copies)	134	111
	(2) Mailed In-County Paid Subscriptions Stated on PS Form 3541 (Include paid distribution above nominal rate, advertiser's proof copies, and exchange copies)		
	(3) Paid Distribution Outside the Mails Including Sales Through Dealers and Carriers, Street Vendors, Counter Sales, and Other Paid Distribution Outside USPS®	51	48
	(4) Paid Distribution by Other Classes Mailed Through the USPS (e.g. First-Class Mail®)		
c. Total Paid Distribution (Sum of 15b (1), (2), (3), and (4))		185	159
d. Free or Nominal Rate Distribution (By Mail and Outside the Mail)	(1) Free or Nominal Rate Outside-County Copies Included on PS Form 3541	59	58
	(2) Free or Nominal Rate In-County Copies Included on PS Form 3541		
	(3) Free or Nominal Rate Copies Mailed at Other Classes Through the USPS (e.g. First-Class Mail)		
	(4) Free or Nominal Rate Distribution Outside the Mail (Carriers or other means)		
e. Total Free or Nominal Rate Distribution (Sum of 15d (1), (2), (3) and (4))		59	58
f. Total Distribution (Sum of 15c and 15e)		244	217
g. Copies not Distributed (See instructions to publishers #4 (page #3))		84	103
h. Total (Sum of 15f and g)		328	320
i. Percent Paid (15c divided by 15f times 100)		75.82%	73.27%

16. Total circulation includes electronic copies. Report circulation on PS Form 3526-X worksheet.

17. Publication of Statement of Ownership
If the publication is a general publication, publication of this statement is required. Will be printed in the December 2014 issue of this publication.

18. Signature and Title of Editor, Publisher, Business Manager, or Owner

Stephen R. Bushing – Inventory Distribution Coordinator

Date
September 14, 2014

I certify that all information furnished on this form is true and complete. I understand that anyone who furnishes false or misleading information on this form or who omits material or information requested on the form may be subject to criminal sanctions (including fines and imprisonment) and/or civil sanctions (including civil penalties).

PS Form 3526, August 2012 (Page 2 of 3)

Moving?

Make sure your subscription moves with you!

To notify us of your new address, find your **Clinics Account Number** (located on your mailing label above your name), and contact customer service at:

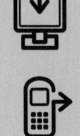

Email: journalscustomerservice-usa@elsevier.com

800-654-2452 (subscribers in the U.S. & Canada)
314-447-8871 (subscribers outside of the U.S. & Canada)

Fax number: 314-447-8029

Elsevier Health Sciences Division
Subscription Customer Service
3251 Riverport Lane
Maryland Heights, MO 63043

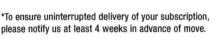

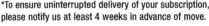

*To ensure uninterrupted delivery of your subscription, please notify us at least 4 weeks in advance of move.

Printed and bound by CPI Group (UK) Ltd, Croydon, CR0 4YY

03/10/2024

01040486-0014